A JOURNEY INTO YIN YOGA

Travis Eliot

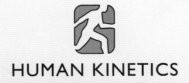

HUMAN KINETICS

Library of Congress Cataloging-in-Publication Data

Names: Eliot, Travis, 1977- author.
Title: A journey into yin yoga / Travis Eliot.
Description: Champaign, IL : Human Kinetics, [2019] | Includes
   bibliographical references. | Description based on print version
   record and CIP data provided by publisher; resource not viewed.
Identifiers: LCCN 2017054032 (print) | LCCN 2017051928 (ebook) | ISBN
   9781492557234 (ebook) | ISBN 9781492557227 (print)
Subjects: LCSH: Yin yoga.
Classification: LCC RA781.73 (print) | LCC RA781.73 .E45 2019 (ebook) | DDC
   613.7/046--dc23
LC record available at https://lccn.loc.gov/2017054032

ISBN: 978-1-4925-5722-7 (print)

This publication is written and published to provide accurate and authoritative information relevant to the subject matter presented. It is published and sold with the understanding that the author and publisher are not engaged in rendering legal, medical, or other professional services by reason of their authorship or publication of this work. If medical or other expert assistance is required, the services of a competent professional person should be sought.

The web addresses cited in this text were current as of March 2018, unless otherwise noted.

Senior Acquisitions Editor: Michelle Maloney; **Developmental Editor:** Laura Pulliam; **Managing Editor:** Ann C. Gindes; **Copyeditor:** Annette Pierce; **Permissions Manager:** Martha Gullo; **Graphic Designer:** Whitney Milburn; **Cover Designer:** Keri Evans; **Cover Design Associate:** Susan Rothermel Allen; **Photographs (cover and interior):** Patricia Pena, © Human Kinetics, unless otherwise noted; **Photo Production Coordinator:** Amy M. Rose; **Photo Production Manager:** Jason Allen; **Senior Art Manager:** Kelly Hendren; **Illustrations:** © Human Kinetics, unless otherwise noted; **Printer:** Versa Press

We thank Astroetic Studios in Los Angeles, California, for assistance in providing the location for the photo shoot for this book.

Human Kinetics books are available at special discounts for bulk purchase. Special editions or book excerpts can also be created to specification. For details, contact the Special Sales Manager at Human Kinetics.

Printed in the United States of America   10 9 8 7 6 5 4 3 2 1

The paper in this book is certified under a sustainable forestry program.

Human Kinetics
P.O. Box 5076
Champaign, IL 61825-5076
Website: www.HumanKinetics.com

In the United States, email info@hkusa.com or call 800-747-4457.
In Canada, email info@hkcanada.com.
In the United Kingdom/Europe, email hk@hkeurope.com.

For information about Human Kinetics' coverage in other areas of the world,
please visit our website: **www.HumanKinetics.com**

E7122

For all my teachers, who have inspired me along the path of yoga and for all students seeking a life of wisdom, balance, and purpose.

CONTENTS

POSE FINDER

Pose Finder *(continued)*

FOREWORD

Yin yoga has exploded in popularity—and for good reason. We would all be well served by adding yin practice to our routines, and Travis' book is an excellent guide for doing just that. Grounded in his personal experience of discovering the potential for yin yoga to heal and strengthen, Travis expertly leads you on a path to this transformational practice.

I first met Travis at a teacher training on yoga medicine, myofascial release, and Chinese medicine I led in Spain, where we were able to connect and share a common interest in the powerful physical effects of these practices. There are many elements that make yin practice so powerful, and the effects on the fascia are one important part. Fascia is a type of connective tissue that creates a three-dimensional scaffolding, interconnected from head to toe to support and protect. Working with the fascia is an important facet of physical healing, regardless of whether that is done by another person (as in massage and other forms of bodywork) or by yourself (as with self-myofascial release methods and yin yoga). Maintaining movement in the fascia is important so that tissues can easily glide past each other and maintain proper hydration, neurologic feedback, pliability, and elasticity.

Tight and restricted fascia can become a source of tension to the rest of the body, producing pain or restricting movement—an all-too-common scenario in our modern times. Although hatha yoga practices can slowly retrain the soft tissue over time, working directly on the fascia with yin yoga can dramatically speed up soft tissue changes and assist in maintaining pliability and strength of the fascia and other connective tissues. Yin yoga is an excellent method of stimulating self-healing, and I use it with a variety of patients, including professional athletes, caregivers, doctors, mothers, and office workers. As a yoga teacher and as a health care provider, I believe this type of yoga practice is still an extremely overlooked aspect of tissue health and overall wellness.

Another aspect that is important to acknowledge is yin yoga's effect on the body's vital energies. Subtle energy, or chi, is often referred to as our *life force* or *energy on the verge of materializing*. A yin practice allows us to be introspective as a way of better adjusting to the fluctuations of this energy in the body. In Chinese medicine, health is depicted as the delicate balance of yin and yang. In this book, Travis' simple explanations of these concepts help the reader understand the importance of balancing these opposing forces of yin and yang in our lives, helping the reader to more easily identify how to amplify health and wellness on a daily basis.

We spend so much of our day-to-day life motored by the adrenaline-fueled sympathetic nervous system (SNS, the fight or flight system) that our parasympathetic nervous system (PNS, the rest and digest system) can weaken and lose its ability to adapt and respond. The more active yoga practices, like vinyasa and ashtanga, feed the SNS-controlled parts of the body, and yin yoga feeds the PNS-controlled parts. If we're only doing physically demanding forms of yoga, we're only accessing half of yoga's potential. Yin helps us create the balance that is essential to our health and wellness.

Yin yoga—as well as pranayama breathing and meditation—helps to tone the precious PNS, allowing us to more easily access the peaceful, quiet, and restorative part of our nature, even in the midst of everyday madness. Taking time to rest in this state serves as a powerful antidote to our stress buildup, helping prevent stress-related health problems; it also helps us develop the skills to minimize our own stress response during challenging moments. Being able to access this stillness during times of emotional strain can improve our relationships, our parenting, and even our careers—and those moments can have a ripple effect throughout our communities.

In this book, Travis highlights the three key points in a yin yoga practice: finding our edge, finding the stillness, and letting time flow. The beyond-time state of meditation he refers to is, in my opinion, where we find a lot of the internal physiological effects happening. This is where the nervous system gets to recalibrate and the effects of the practice are magnified. The stillness is essential—not only to relax the muscles but also to target the deeper connective tissue and create space for the nervous system to soak up the effects and translate them to the rest of the body. Yin yoga gives us permission to completely relax and to surrender to a practice that gives our body the space it needs to rest, recover, and heal—allowing connective tissues to become stronger and the internal body to become more resilient. The simplicity we find in the stillness and silence of yin practice just might be the most potent medicine for our modern lives.

This book gives you the tools you need to begin this potent practice and reap the benefits for many years to come. In this book, you have access to instruction and inspiration from a world-renowned teacher who can help you find your path to strength of body and mind. You are in good hands with Travis as your yin yoga guide.

—Tiffany Cruikshank, LAc, MAOM, founder of Yoga Medicine

PREFACE

Naturally, when you discover something amazing, you want to share it with as many people as possible. After getting hit by a car as a pedestrian, I was left injured, scared, and feeling down—that is, until I found yin yoga. It was life changing!

As a teacher, I started incorporating yin yoga at the end of my power yoga classes in Santa Monica. We called the class Yoga Stretch because back then, yin classes were extremely rare. People loved it! I was surprised, because I thought people would be bored. I mean, who wants to sit around doing nothing, discovering uncomfortable places in the body, and dealing with the challenging mental component? Plus, if you've been running away from something, it will be able to catch up with you when you become still. This can be challenging because you will need to confront it. In yin yoga, stillness helps you to face these things and triggers physical, emotional, and spiritual processes that can holistically improve your health. Fortunately, the students in my first yin class got it, and the class quickly became popular among a wide range of people.

From there, I started teaching yin yoga in teacher trainings and retreats, and although it wasn't love at first sight for a lot of people, I did notice that it seemed to fill a void. Students reported to me that their longstanding injuries were starting to heal, their sleep improved immensely, their bodies became more flexible, their stress levels dropped, and most important, they began to notice positive benefits in their relationships and careers.

I filmed yin yoga practices for *The Ultimate Yogi* and *Yoga 30 for 30* programs, and that spread the power of yin to students in more than 40 countries worldwide. All sorts of people were introduced to yin for the first time. Professional athletes, celebrities, entertainers, business executives, health care practitioners, teachers, and lawyers reached out, sharing how yin yoga was changing their lives.

Now more than ever, people need yin yoga to balance the fast pace of modern life. Moving at such a hurried and frenetic pace can lead to high levels of stress, illness, and depression and is not sustainable. At some point, you have to ease your foot off the pedal and just let the engine idle. Better yet, just switch the engine off. Otherwise the engine will blow.

Yin yoga provides us an opportunity to slow down, to go within, and to go deep. Some cultures call it the sacred pause. It's within that pause, or moment of stillness, that we come back to our inner most essence. By dropping into this stillness, we find our center. When we are centered, things don't throw us out of balance so easily. We find that we are able to move through the world, even in all of its challenges, with more grace, steadiness, and nobility.

Yin yoga is sometimes called the fountain of youth. As people grow older, their bodies lose flexibility, tension increases, circulation is inhibited, and tissues begin to atrophy and deteriorate. Yin yoga can stop or even reverse this process greatly, thereby slowing the aging process. In yin yoga, we can activate deeper connective tissues through long, deep stretching that exerts positive pressure on them. This sets into motion a chain of events in which the body heals the collagen and elastin fibers of the connective tissues, making them stronger and more durable.

The Taoists drew much inspiration from nature. One example of this is the Shaolin fighting monks that were named after the Shaolin tree. When fierce storms blew through their area, often the only trees left standing were the Shaolin trees. This was because of both their strength and their suppleness. Without suppleness in the body and mind, there's a good chance that at some point you will snap. Yin yoga helps to cultivate flexibility and adaptability within all aspects of your life so that you are ready for whatever comes your way!

ACKNOWLEDGMENTS AND BOWS OF GRATITUDE

To Lauren Eckstrom, my wife, who loves and inspires me every day. Thank you for keeping me on course when 85 pages were lost into the mysterious void of the digital world.

To Etan Boritzer, a friend, who selflessly guided me into the intricate world of book publishing.

To Michelle Maloney, my acquisitions editor, who believed in this book from day one.

To Laura Pulliam, my developmental editor, who helped shape my manuscript so that it would flow like the Tao.

To Patricia Pena, my photographer, for your cinematic eye.

To Bryan Kest, Govind Das, Stic, A.J. Pollock, Dr. Jeremy Brook, Dr. Adam Griffin, Dr. Michael Galitzer, Flo Master, Desi Bartlett, Matt Kahrs, and Dana Byerlee for sharing their knowledge and inspiration.

To the pioneers and senior teachers of yin yoga, Master Cho, Paulie Zink, Paul Grilley, Sarah Powers, and Bernie Clark.

To my meditation and dharma teachers, Jack Kornfield and Tara Brach.

To my mom, Charlotte Smith, for planting the seeds of awakening in me at an early age.

To my dad, John Smith, for teaching me that anything is possible.

To my kids, Lantana and Bodhi, for teaching me about true love.

To the lady who hit me with her car and sent me down this path; if it hadn't been for you, this book wouldn't exist.

INTRODUCTION

In 2004, and I was in downtown Los Angeles walking to my car after attending a meeting. It was a typical sunny, warm afternoon in Southern California. My meeting went well and I was eager to get to my car and get some food. I arrived on the corner of a busy intersection and waited for the pedestrian signal. Although I was alone on my side of the intersection, there were a couple of people on the opposite side. One was a businessman in a light-gray suit, and the other was a student jamming out to music with his headphones on.

My car stereo had a detachable faceplate you could remove to prevent a thief from stealing the stereo, and I had stuffed this plate into the outer pocket of my meeting planner. After the light signaled me to go, I started across the street. I remember that after taking several steps, I was still contemplating where to get food. At that moment, out of the corner of my eye, I saw a large object coming straight at me. It was a car, and it was coming fast!

My mind raced at lightning speed, assessing its survival options. The car was coming at me way too quickly for me to jump forward. Jumping back also wasn't an option. Going to the side would have been even worse. The bumper would nail me right at the knees, most likely buckling me over and slamming my body and head into the pavement.

So, what do you do when all your options look pretty bleak? You jump! You jump as fast as possible, because it's do or die. So that's what I did: My brain issued its command, flooded me with a tsunami of adrenaline, and I jumped straight up. About this time, the driver finally noticed me and slammed on the brakes, but it was too late. As I started to float down from my Michael Jordanesque jump, the car moved under me, and I crashed into the windshield with a sound so loud that people blocks away heard the collision. All of a sudden, I was coasting through the air for what seemed like an eternity. I remember distinctly noticing the rich blue sky and the bright golden sun as I rose into the air.

However, in an instant this poetic moment was shattered when I came crashing down. The thing was, though, I magically came down hard on both feet. There I was, miraculously standing in the middle of a busy intersection in the middle of downtown Los Angeles, thinking "What the hell just happened?!" The driver was in total shock. In slow motion, I could see the businessman and the student running over to me. My stereo faceplate was somehow wedged under the car's windshield wiper blade. And my meeting planner had ended up inside the car. Some things even physics can't explain.

As the witnesses helped me to the sidewalk, I heard sirens approaching. Someone in an office building down the street had heard the crash and called 911. After the paramedics checked me out, the police filed a report and reality started to sink in. I had narrowly escaped, with just some minor gashes and a limp, what could have been a life-changing, devastating accident. I declined to go to the hospital, and after I signed some papers, the paramedics cleared me to leave.

I hobbled back to my car, and every time I stepped onto my right foot, my knee gave out. This condition continued for many months. The injury continued to bother me when I walked, and jogging was definitely out of the question. I was resigned to the fact that my joy for running was now a thing of the past.

Ten years after my accident, I was in Costa Rica conducting an international Holistic Yoga Flow teacher training. Once a year, for the past three years, my wife Lauren and I invite people from all over the world to join us for a three-week intensive teacher training. It includes 10 hours a day of yoga practice, meditation, lectures, workshops, homework, and teaching practice for 21 days straight.

Lauren teaches half the day, and then I teach the other half. The retreat center that particular year was at the Costa Rica Yoga Spa, located up in the hills of Nosara. This majestic part of the country is nestled between the Montana and Nosara rivers, with breathtaking views of Costa Rica's Gold Coast of Guanacaste.

On our last full day of the training I decided to do a trail run through the jungle, as I had done many times over the last weeks. But this time felt different. I found myself drenched in sweat, my heart thundering, and at times it felt like it could explode out my chest. I don't mean that in a dangerous way; I mean it in the best possible way. I had never felt so invigorated, awake, clear, inspired, and full to the brim with vitality. My body felt invincible, like I was a superhero! My mind felt sharp and my heart radiantly alive. It was one of those rare moments that's truly a peak experience.

As I continued to run through the hills, not one soul was in sight. In fact, I hadn't seen another person for well over three hours. But there had been an abundance of other life forms. Periodically, I heard a big rumble coming from the trees. It almost sounded like a monster from a child's bedtime story. In this case, though, it was howler monkeys, famous in this part of the country. They move as a tribe through the trees, rummaging for their favorite food. Although their howl is quite intimidating, they keep to themselves and are harmless. I also saw some shy and much more rare spider monkeys, and I stopped briefly to exchange eye contact with one in particular. It looked nervous, but I did my best to communicate with my eyes that I came in respect and peace. Then it went along its way, and I continued my run. At that point in the run, I had set a new personal record, having covered more than 14 miles (23.5 km) with some dramatic total elevation gains and all without a bite of food or a drop of water.

Something strange was happening. I felt like I could keep running forever; I didn't want to stop. Not only did my physical body feel superhuman, but I also felt as if my spirit had been freed from a cage. I could feel the otherworldly spirit of the jungle. The plants, trees, rocks, mountains, water, insects, animals, sky, and sun were all connected. As the boundaries of my body seemed to fade away and the walls of my mind seemed to blur, I could feel one with all. I was having a life-changing experience. It's what the yogis call moksha, or the Taoists call nirvana. I'll never forget that transcendental run through the Costa Rican jungle.

The interesting thing is, yin yoga is what allowed me to run again even though I never thought it would be possible. Months after the accident, I had discovered yin yoga. It's crazy how you can look back at certain moments in life and realize how one event can shift your entire future. For me, this was finding the *Yin Yoga* DVD with Paul Grilley. I had done lots of power yoga and vinyasa classes, but this was my first introduction to this other style of yoga. Paul Grilley's DVD contained multiple practices you could do, and it also came with an educational discourse on the science of yin.

I also attended live classes with Bryan Kest in Santa Monica, who always included a pose in his sequence in which you bring your knees together, spread your feet wider than your hips, and sit between the ankles. In hatha yoga it's called hero pose or virasana. Bryan must have loved this pose because he would do it two or three times in every class. At first it was painful, very painful. But it was the good pain, and Bryan always reminded us not to push too far. He also had a legendary sequence he sometimes taught called long, slow, and deep, or more famously, LSD. Although he didn't call it yin, it definitely was. LSD is a seamless floor series of postures held for long periods and could often last for two and a half to three hours. At the end of those classes, I felt reborn!

Within just a few weeks of practicing yin yoga with Paul and Bryan, my knee had completely healed, and not only did my knee feel better, but actually my whole body felt incredible. Recently, I set a new personal record running a full marathon through the mountains. At some point, I even hope to run an ultramarathon of more than 50 miles (80 km).

So how did this happen? How was I able to go from barely walking to running long distances? It's simple. It was yin yoga. Yin yoga became an integral component of my personal path and practice. As you will see in the following pages, yin yoga has many layers. Yes, it's physical, but it's much more than that, and to neglect that would be a huge irresponsibility on my part. So, my aim in this book is to give you my all. My hope is that you will be inspired to use yin yoga as way to align with the best version of yourself.

We start by covering the background of yoga and the compelling history of how yin yoga came to be. We will also explore the philosophy of Taoism and how it relates to yin yoga. From a yoga perspective, we will take a look at the more subtle energetic aspects of the body. The "meat and potatoes" of the book details the science of what happens when we do a yin practice. We will also explore more than 50 yin postures and counter stretches, explaining their benefits, contraindications, alignment points, modifications, and their suggested duration. The book concludes with chapters on special breathing exercises and meditations. I've also included 5 important yang sequences, and 10 thematic yin sequences that students can do at home and teachers can draw from for their own classes. What's mine is yours. Lastly, we finish our journey together with final thoughts of "yinspiration"!

My intention is that this book provides much more than a textbook experience. Throughout these pages are stories, quotes, and conversations with experts to enhance the teachings. My hope is that your learning experience will be exciting and enjoyable. I am both honored and excited to be your guide as we now journey into this wonderful world of yin yoga!

Travis Eliot
Los Angeles
June 2017

CHAPTER 1
ORIGINS OF YOGA

"The journey of a thousand miles begins with a single step."

—Lao Tzu

Often in the Western world when you mention the word yoga, what pops into mind is an image of a person doing a yoga posture. You might picture somebody doing a down dog or handstand or some fancy posture where he or she is tied up in a knot, looking like a pretzel. The truth of the matter is that yoga is so much more than just poses.

Yoga comes from the Sanskrit root word, *yuj*, which means to yoke or to unite. So, what exactly is uniting? Well, it can be many things. A farmer 100 years ago might have united a plow with an ox to help plow the field. When two people get married, you could say that's yoga. Vinyasa yoga students might unite their breath with movement to induce a flow. People who meditate might unite their focus with a mantra or an affirmation. Spiritual people might dedicate their entire lives to uniting themselves with a higher power through every thought, word, or action. In fact, this latter example is where yoga all began.

EIGHT LIMBS OF YOGA

The original forms of yoga date back many thousands of years. The earliest known writings of yoga can be found in ancient spiritual texts called the **Vedas** that date back from 1700 BCE to 1100 BCE. The Vedas are sacred scriptures from India. Veda comes from the root *vid*, to know. The Vedas are revealed knowledge given to humanity at the dawn of time. They exist in four collections: Rig, Sama, Yajur, and Atharva. The Rig Veda is the oldest. Born of the Vedas are the Upanishads. Although parts of the Vedas define the religion of a certain culture, the Upanishads are considered to be universal. It is commonly believed that the Upanishads are as relevant to the world today as they were to India 5,000 years ago.

The traditional style of yoga was called raja yoga. **Raja yoga** is known as royal yoga or classical yoga and focuses on meditation and contemplation. It is known as the royal yoga because the royal families of India invited sages, or spiritual masters, to teach the royal family about yoga. In the beginning, yoga had nothing to do with the physical and everything to do with the science of the mind.

Centuries later, around 200 to 400 CE, a person named **Patanjali** systemized this classical form of raja yoga into the eight limbs of yoga. The eight limbs of yoga consist of a series of sutras that pack a powerful punch of information that is short and to the point. Each sutra is inclusive of all people regardless of age, gender, ethnicity, or religious belief. The eight limbs of yoga provide a road map for reaching the peak human experience in which a person is liberated, enlightened, and awakened!

"The second you stepped into this world of existence a ladder was placed before you to help you escape it." —Rumi

Let's explore a brief overview of Patanjali's system. Like the quote from the poet Rumi, let's start at the bottom of the ladder and work our way up. We begin with Yama.

Limb One: Yamas, or Awakened Qualities

Yama refers to ethics, integrity, and how we practice yoga off of our mats in relation to others. The five yamas are ahimsa, satya, asteya, brahmacharya, and aparigraha.

Ahimsa, or Nonviolence

Life is incredibly sacred. It is through being alive that we all have the capacity to love, to serve, and to lift each other up. When we inflict violence against ourselves or others, we are violating that potential.

Nonviolence, or **ahisma**, begins with our actions. On one level, this is the easiest stage to achieve—not physically hurting others. Once we eradicate violent behavior, we must eliminate violence from our speech. Verbal abuse has the potential to be just as damaging as physical abuse and sometimes even more so. The final stage, and the hardest to achieve, is to remove violence from our minds and to be diligent with our thoughts. This takes a lot of practice because of the complexity of our minds.

Fortunately, Patanjali had a technique called pratipaksha bhavana, which teaches us to spin a negative thought into a positive one. It's important to understand that we will experience anger and rage; the key is to harness these powerful emotions and transform them for a higher good. Two great examples of people who mastered this practice are Mahatma Gandhi and an activist he inspired, Dr. Martin Luther King Jr. Both were able to radically effect positive change. Just like these great figures, we all have the ability through nonviolence to unlock infinite reserves of compassion and love.

Satya, or Truthfulness

Thomas Jefferson said, "Honesty is the first chapter in the book of wisdom." When we violate truth by telling lies—no matter how big or small—we pollute our minds. And when our minds become murky, we are imprisoned within our self-created confusion. This is why you hear the expression "The truth will set you free." By aligning our speech and actions with truthfulness, or **satya**, we stand on invincible ground. Speaking the truth can sometimes be difficult, but it always carries us down the path of grace and nobility.

Asteya, or Nonstealing

Stealing is taking something from someone who does not freely give it. This can apply to personal possessions, money, and land, but it can also apply to another person's time and energy. In relationships or in business, it's important to know how to establish boundaries with certain people—some folks can be needy and hijack our attention. It is said that a person firmly committed against stealing, or committed to **asteya**, will receive a steady stream of material and spiritual wealth. One who feels abundance also attracts abundance; the person no longer chases after opportunities because opportunities come chasing after the person. It is a beautiful moment along the yoga path when you realize that everything you want already exists within.

Brahmacharya, or Celibacy

In ancient times, yogis renounced all forms of sexual activity, believing that they could use the sexual energy they harnessed to become spiritually enlightened. Although this practice might work well for a person isolated in a forest or a cave, it's more difficult when you are out in the world dealing with families, relationships, and careers.

Another issue that complicates the strict definition of celibacy, or **brahmacharya**, is that repressing sexual energy can lead to destructive acts, such as disrespecting ourselves or someone else, which can unleash anger, jealousy, and negativity. At the same time, when combined with love, physical intimacy can support us along our spiritual path. So, celibacy as part of brahmacharya today means using sexual energy in a way that is moderate and respectful.

Aparigraha, or Nongrasping

In the yogic tradition, it is believed that that grasping or developing an attachment to something or someone causes suffering. We've all seen a toddler having a meltdown in a store when their parent wouldn't buy them a toy or a piece of candy. The more attached this child is to what they want, the more they suffer.

For adults, it's the same thing. Do you possess your possessions or do they possess you? Are you holding onto the past? It's important to yield to the fact that everything is in a constant state of flux and change. When we resist change, or try to latch onto something that's temporary, we create tremendous inner conflict and suffering. This self-created stress can greatly detract from our health and well-being. Nongrasping, or **aparigraha**, also refers to taking only what we need and no more. Can you imagine every person, corporation, and country respecting this? Our planet would be in a much healthier state. As Gandhi has said, "There is enough for everyone's need, but not enough for everyone's greed."

Limb Two: Niyama, or Codes for Noble Living

Niyama deals with self-discipline and spiritual practices in relationship to ourselves. The five niyamas are saucha, santosha, tapas, svadhyaya, and ishvara pranidhana.

Saucha, or Purity

Purity, or **saucha**, can start in external spaces such as the home, car, or office. In the Chinese tradition, this is called feng shui, and in yoga it is called vastu. The idea in both systems is that clean, open spaces allow room for energy to flow, which increases productivity, creativity, and even happiness.

You've probably spent a long Saturday afternoon cleaning out a desk, a closet, or a room and then felt so good when you were finally done. This is an example of saucha. Taking it a step further, we should also make sure that our yoga and meditation space is clean and pure and make sure that our bodies are pure, too. By eating nutritious, wholesome food free of chemicals and preservatives, we can help our bodies and brains function in their optimal states. The senses will therefore be sharpened and our relationship with the outer world heightened. We should be conscious of what we feed our senses. For example, right before going to bed is probably not the best time to indulge in TV that is highly agitating and violent. Instead, we should feed our minds material that is positive, inspiring, and uplifting.

Santosha, or Contentment

Contentment, or **santosha**, is about maintaining equanimity through all of life's ups and downs. It also can be a powerful state of mind in which you constantly feel grateful for all of the blessings that exist in your life.

You have the choice to move through life reflecting on all that you have or ruminating on what you don't. Constantly complaining about what you don't have creates a reality of deficiency and emptiness, which can be a miserable way to live. On the flip side, dwelling in a state of gratitude for what you do have creates a state of fullness, richness, and abundance.

It's possible to create such a strong momentum of abundance that all sorts of amazing opportunities will fly into your life. However, as a human being, you face challenges big and small each and every day. It's important in the midst of difficulties to search for the silver lining. Everything happens for a good reason, even though it can be difficult to see it in the midst of the experience.

Also, contentment should never be confused with complacency. If you are in a harmful or hurtful situation, you should move out of that situation as quickly as possible. The key is to move through the challenge with equanimity.

Tapas, or Purification

The definition of **tapas** is to burn. Just as placing gold into a fire burns away the impurities or placing a magnifying glass so that the sun shines through it and ignites a fire, we can create a positive burn within ourselves.

To engage in tapas, you must be highly disciplined. Tapas can take many forms. On a physical level, you could participate in a juice fast for five days. If you've done this, you know that it isn't easy: You must move through the withdrawal symptoms such as intense cravings for sugar, caffeine, and food. Through this act you are taking steps to affect your wellness.

Another form of tapas is to take a vow of silence for a certain amount of time. Being completely silent is an intense experience, but this is an effective way to purify your speech and clearly illuminate the things you might say that are negative. Another great example of tapas is meditation. Perhaps you sit with your eyes closed and silently repeat a mantra. If you're like most people, you are bombarded with distracting thoughts that pull you away from the mantra. But each time you return to the repetition, you are helping to purify your mind, even if it feels daunting to try to burn away the unnecessary thoughts. Through discipline and by staying aligned with your tapas, you have the potential to invoke powerful stages of transformation.

Svadhyaya, or Self-Study

The moment we stop growing is the moment we stop living. It is within our nature to keep learning and expanding, and we must have the humility to know that we don't know it all. We must stay ferocious within our quest to learn more.

Self-study, or **svadhyaya**, is how we achieve this. As children, we constantly study, but we often slow down or stop altogether when we become adults with jobs and new responsibilities. Before we know it, we can become mindless drones trudging through our jobs and our lives. But life is more than just surviving—it's about thriving!

Self-study ignites an inner passion that makes life extraordinary. So, whether it's enrolling in a yoga teacher training program, watching an inspiring documentary, reading a spiritual text, or studying this book, find time every day for self-study.

Ishvara Pranidhana, or Celebration of the Divine

Celebration of the divine, also known as **ishvara pranidhana**, is also a celebration of spirit. It is revering a force that is much bigger than our own limited self. Cultures throughout history have accomplished this through song, dance, poetry, art, worship, festivals, and spending time in nature.

Devoting ourselves to a higher power gives us perspective. We learn not to worry about unimportant details. We transcend out of isolation and ascend into a connectedness with the pulse of the universe at large. We realize that although things appear separate on a superficial level, on a deeper level everything is one. As we'll see later in our journey, this is the secret of connection that the Taoists had discovered. Not only do we start to see the divine within us, but we also see it in all people and all life forms. We realize that everything we think, say, and do affects not only our inner world but also the outer world. Instead of being selfish, we become selfless. We tap into a permanent state of peace, knowing that the secret to living is giving. By giving to others, we give immeasurably back to ourselves.

Limb Three: Asana, or Pose

Asana is the physical posture; this is the limb of yoga that the majority of us are most familiar with. One definition of asana is to sit quietly within. But if many of the asanas are standing postures, why did the yogis state it this way? They weren't talking about the physical postures, but about something more subtle: a state of mind that is calm, steady, and at ease.

More important than *what we do* on our mats is *how we do what we do*. Yoga teaches us that we can bring the asana mind state into our relationships, careers, lovemaking, and chores—even to running errands and the other mundane parts of life.

Through asana we dissolve tensions, build strength, eliminate toxins, increase mobility, and circulate freshly oxygenated blood throughout the entire body. Physical yoga helps us to not only become strong like steel but also light like a feather. It also helps boost our immune system. It's nearly guaranteed that we'll flourish when our immune system is robust. And physical practice releases the natural feel-good stimulants, such as endorphins and serotonin. When we practice a strong pose such as warrior II, we often feel an energy of deep strength. When we feel this strength, it supports us throughout the day so that we are ready for whatever comes our way. We know that we have the strength and power to handle whatever the universe brings us.

Because much of our culture is dominated by vanity and aesthetics, it's easy to get stuck in this limb. Being an advanced yogi doesn't mean that you can do arm balances and inversions like they are circus tricks. What good is being able to balance upside down if you can't bring compassion and love into the world? In fact, advanced postures often become a trap for people's egos. It's easy to compete and compare your poses to those of others. But remember comparison is the thief of joy. Simply think of a pose as a means to an end, shifting you from a state of doing into a state of being. The pose is a means for you to ascend to your higher self and help you sit in meditation for longer periods of time.

Limb Four: Pranayama, or Breath Control

Pranayama is the expansion of life force through breathing exercises. When you shape your breath, you shape your mind. The last time you were frustrated, angry, scared, or anxious, what happened to your breath? It probably became restricted, choppy, and erratic. How about when you were happy and centered? Most likely, your breath was even, smooth, and rhythmic. So, we know that breath and the mental state are deeply connected.

Pranayama should always be learned from a qualified instructor, and just like physical yoga, it should be performed without straining. The goal is not to see how long you can hold your breath, although over time you will notice breath retention taking less effort. Instead, the objective is to master the flow of the breath. The breath is the foundation of the physical practice. Make the breath the focus and from there everything will fall into place. The power of the breath will lead you to the posture's sweet spot with ease.

When you focus on the breath, you can give gratitude for its support and nourishment. With each inhalation, you breathe vitality into your being, and with each exhalation, you surrender everything that is no longer serving you. The gift of breath is the gift of life.

Limb Five: Pratyahara, or Sense Control

Pratyahara is the control of or withdrawal from the five senses. Throughout our lives, the senses of touch, taste, sight, hearing, and smell provide information to our brains. When practicing pratyahara, we shut off the external flow of data, giving ourselves the opportunity to retreat within. Just like astronauts explore outer space, yogis investigate the inner space.

If we are always looking outside of ourselves, how will we ever really know who we are, what we are made of, why we are here, and what we came here to do? Some people are afraid of looking within, frightened of what they might discover. Certainly, anything that you've been avoiding or running away from will finally have an opportunity to present itself while you practice pratyahara. It is for these moments that we practice warrior poses, so that we have the courage to face our inner demons. These inner demons are part of what makes us human, and we must learn to somehow love that aspect of ourselves if we are to free ourselves from their grasp. The things we resist persist, and we are able to move through the things we embrace with grace.

Often in yoga, we use the metaphor of a person driving a chariot to illustrate the role of the senses. The five senses are like five horses, the chariot represents the body, and the driver represents the mind. Sadly, in many instances, the five senses, or horses, run wild and inevitably lead the person and the chariot off a cliff. However, when we take command of our senses, we are able to steer ourselves down the path of health, integrity, and joy. This stage can take a significant amount of time to master, but it's a key turning point into the final stages of fully experiencing the eight limbs of yoga.

Limb Six: Dharana, or Focus and Concentration

Dharana, which means focus or concentration, is the first stage of meditation. Focus, like muscle, becomes stronger the more you use it. In this case, the "muscle" exists within your brain. The brain is composed of neural branches that create patterns in the way you think, speak, and act. Through **neuroplasticity**, which is the ability to change the neural pathways through behavior, you are able to mold or rewire your brain. Through dharana, you can reinforce certain neural connections, giving you the power to set up a brain system that will help you achieve the type of life you want to live.

When practicing dharana, you can focus on many different things. You can focus on an audible or silent mantra, an affirmation, a candle flame, a picture, a prayer, your breath, a sensation, or just about anything else. More important than what you focus on, though, is the actual act of focusing.

Often when you sit down and begin to focus, the mind starts to wander. Perhaps you recall a recent conversation, remember something to add to your to-do list, or come up with an amazing idea. When you notice the distraction, gently bring the mind back to the object of focus. It's possible that you may spend the entire time chasing your mind. The mind secretes thoughts like the salivary glands secrete saliva. In fact, in his book *destressifying*, Davidji writes, "…our mind processes 60,000 to 80,000 thoughts throughout the 1,440 minutes in every 24-hour day. That's a thought every 1.2 seconds" (2015, 83). So, you won't try to stop the thoughts, but rather try to direct them. Don't get discouraged, and know that each time you bring your mind back, you've completed an exercise inside your brain. Would you expect your chest and arms to become well developed after a few push-ups? Of course not! Just as with physical training, with dharana, it takes hundreds, even thousands, of repetitions to notice a difference.

Building the muscle of concentration uses the same process. The keys are patience and consistency. Eventually, your focus will become so strong that it penetrates like a laser beam through all distraction.

Limb Seven: Dhyana, or Meditation

Dhyana is meditation, or total absorption into the object that is being focused on. What's the difference between dharana and dhyana? Dharana requires effort. It's like knocking on the door of dhyana. You can't force your way into a state of dhyana; you must be invited in. You could call this invitation an act of grace.

Imagine you are sitting down to meditate and your chosen object is a candle flame. The practice of gazing at the flame is called **tradak**. While gazing at the flame, you notice your mind wandering. Like a dedicated yogi, you release the distraction and resume concentrating on the flame. Now, you are in the state of dharana. Then, after some time, your mind begins to settle and all of a sudden you've slipped into a state in which there is no longer a separation between you, the observer, and the flame, which is the object. You've become one with the object. This is dhyana.

A good gauge for knowing whether you have accessed dhyana is if time seems to fly by. If you are thinking, "When is this meditation going to be done?" you are still in the limb of dharana. Conversely, if you think, "I can't believe how fast the time flew by!" then most likely you were in dhyana. In a state of meditation, you transcend time, body, place, and space.

Because it's out of your control whether you shift into dhyana or not, it's important to remain detached. Some days it will happen and other days it won't. All you can do is keep showing up on your meditation cushion. Just like practicing a musical instrument, it's much better to do a little meditation every day than to do a lot once a week.

Limb Eight: Samadhi, or Absolute Oneness

Samadhi is the source of all yoga. It's difficult to describe in words because it is a state that exists beyond the realm of labels, ideas, and forms. This might be why poetry and music were created; they help people experience a glimpse of samadhi. In samadhi, the sense of I dissolves, and you become one with all creation. You reunite with the place from which you were born, and the place you will one day dissolve into, like a tiny drop of rain falling into an infinite ocean of stillness.

A yogi who has a samadhi experience realizes that our humanity consists of more than the obvious characteristics. There is more than our skin color, age, gender, ethnicity, and occupation. In a state of samadhi, we see through the illusionary veil of separateness and know that we are all one.

All of the other limbs are in preparation for samadhi. Reaching samadhi is like summiting a mountain top. It is said that when just one person reaches samadhi, it benefits all humanity. But as incredible as samadhi is, you still must function within the world. After enlightenment and the big awakening, you still have to wash laundry, do your taxes, and remember your Social Security number. You must come down from the mountain and return to the valley. As you descend, though, you bring the awakening with you. You must bring love where there is anger, joy where there is sadness, health where there is disease, forgiveness where there is resentment, peace where there is chaos, and light where there is darkness.

The eight limbs of yoga are meant to serve as a guide. It's easy to get lost and allow ourselves to be pulled away from our path, the path that is in alignment with our greatest potential. The farther that we move away from this path, the greater our suffering becomes. The closer that we stay to this path, the happier, healthier, and more peaceful we will be. Patanjali and all the yogis before him were gracious enough to compile this information into an easy-to-follow universal system that was powerful thousands of years ago, is powerful today, and will be powerful for centuries to come.

TRADITIONAL PATHS OF YOGA

As mentioned earlier, the eight limbs of yoga from Patanjali were born from the path of raja yoga. I say path intentionally because that's what it is. It's a path that you can follow, and through dedication and persistence, you will eventually reach the summit of human experience, which is to become enlightened. Another word we could use is *awakened,* as we wake up to our true highest nature. Like the state of samadhi, we transcend the small self and connect to the big Self.

Outside of raja yoga, which emphasizes the science of the mind through meditation, are other paths that can take you to the summit of human consciousness. Although they may be different, they will get you to the same place. Yoga teaches that you are your own master, and you walk the path that feels right for you. We are all different and unique. In fact, in the history of humanity, there has never been a person quite like you.

The other traditional paths besides raja yoga include jnana yoga, karma yoga, bhakti yoga, and hatha yoga. Let's explore these other styles.

Jnana Yoga

Jnana yoga is the yoga of knowledge. It provides the path of self-realization through both a mental and an experiential understanding. It's one thing to understand something intellectually, but a whole other thing to know something from direct experience.

The Buddha (Siddhartha Gautama, 563 BCE – 483 BCE) might be considered one of the most powerful jnana yogis in history. He lived a life of discipline and high principles, practicing peacefulness, truthfulness, generosity, and celibacy and refraining from all intoxicants. He learned various meditation techniques from contemporary masters, and he trained his mind to reach extremely deep states of concentration. However, he still felt something was missing. It wasn't until a fateful day and night when he took his seat with an unshakable determination to awaken himself that he finally found everything he had been seeking. He became fully liberated from delusion, greed, and hatred, and it all happened through his own direct experience.

After many years of intense spiritual practice, the Buddha still hadn't become fully awakened. At the age of 35, he decided to sit under a Bodhi tree (the tree of knowledge) until he became completely awakened. By awakened, we mean to come out of the delusions that most of us live in. As the Buddhist scriptures state, The Buddha sat in a crossed-legged meditative posture, closed his eyes, and began to focus his mind on the natural rhythm of the breath. As his mind became more concentrated, his awareness of Reality deepened until he experienced his entire being as a constant flow of sensations. Although the muscles and bones of the body appear on one level to be dense, concrete, and hard, on a deeper subatomic level, everything is pure energy made of **kalapas**, the smallest subatomic particles of physical matter. The Buddha realized these subatomic particles that he was feeling flowing through his body were also what made up his thoughts and feelings; in fact, his entire mind.

As his experience deepened during the days he sat beneath the Bodhi tree, The Buddha realized directly that all the matter throughout the universe was a great eternal flow of trillions of these kalapas. His great awakening then expanded into the realization that the endless flow of kalapas was the cause of impermanence (anicca) of all phenomena. The Buddha's freedom thus came about from opening his mind to knowing directly the universal laws of nature. For 45 years after his awakening, The Buddha taught countless people his meditation technique known as **vipassana**, which means insight, or to see things as they really are. The Buddha's teachings empowered people to understand that the wisdom and knowledge he had attained could also be achieved through their direct experience in meditation.

Albert Einstein is a great example of a person who acted as a modern day jnana yogi. He used the instrument of the mind to revolutionize science through his direct experience. In fact, he said, "Information is not knowledge. The only source of knowledge is experience." He unlocked some of the greatest mysteries of the universe through the power of his mind. Einstein did this with a laser-like focus and heightened concentration, similar to meditation, that revealed to him, through direct experiences, certain hidden laws of nature. His findings would change the course of modern-day science as we know it. So, we can see with these historical examples, that in jnana yoga one uses the power of the mind to directly experience the true nature of reality at the subtlest levels. And it is these direct experiences that lead one to enlightenment, a state wherein we gain real knowledge of the deepest truths of existence.

Karma Yoga

Sir Isaac Newton's Third Law of Motion states for every action, there is an equal and opposite reaction. Karma is a figurative Third Law of Motion. The way you treat people affects how they react and treat you in return. How you take care of your body affects how it functions for you, and thinking positively attracts positivity to you.

Karma yoga is the path of using thoughts, speech, and actions in ways that are of service to others. Naturally, when we give to others, we also receive. It's a two-way street. The more generous and kind to others we are, the happier we will be. Mother Teresa is a great example of someone whose actions were in line with a karma yogi. She dedicated her entire existence to taking care of the sick and the poor. A true karma yogi gives without expecting anything in return. Many people give, but they might expect to be acknowledged or that the favor will be returned down the road. This isn't within the true spirit of generosity.

When we give to others with a pure heart, it begins to awaken something within us that is truly magnificent. The point of all forms of yoga is to attune to the interconnectedness of life. When we realize that everything we think, say, and do has an impact on us and the world around us, we can tap into the real power of karma yoga.

Bhakti Yoga

Bhakti yoga is the path of love and devotion. This is where we devote ourselves emotionally to God, spirit, and the divine. This can be accomplished through music, dance, art, and poetry. Like the other paths of yoga, the point in bhakti yoga is to take ourselves beyond our limited selves and back to our true eternal nature.

Since I started practicing yoga I have always felt a real affinity with bhakti yoga, especially the musical aspects of the path. One example of this is kirtan, which came from India and has exploded in popularity at yoga studios through the western world. Kirtan is a musical experience in which a singer leads a music group. The singer calls out a mantra and the audience sings the mantra back. Think about the last music concert you went to. Chances are there was a moment when the lead singer sang something, and then the entire auditorium sang it back, and it was electrifying. Perhaps this was even the highlight of the whole show.

This is how kirtan is the entire time. It's as if you are a part of the band and a cocreator of the music. Traditionally, kirtan uses Sanskrit mantras and names of God. Just like a yoga pose purifies the body, a mantra purifies the mind and the heart. As these become purified, our natural qualities of compassion, forgiveness, and love become fully expressed. In the end, love is the essence of life. On two occasions I have had a brush with death. In both instances, when confronted with my death, I didn't think about anything material or physical. I didn't think about my car, favorite shoes, job, or money. I thought about all the people I loved in my life and all the people that had demonstrated their love to me.

Anytime you create music or art for God, you are engaging in bhakti yoga. Love and devotion give you wings to take flight above and beyond the ego and into a boundless and infinite place. From this place, you have the immediate potential to transform yourself, your family, your community, and the world. Let there be love.

Hatha Yoga

In India, the most common form of yoga is bhakti. In the West, the most common form is **hatha yoga**. Hatha means sun and moon; you could also say yang and yin. It is about finding the balance between these two opposing forces of nature.

Hatha yoga began to flourish around the 10th century CE as a way to support yogis' meditation practices through the use of asanas (postures) and breathing techniques (pranayama). One of the main texts from this tradition is the *Hatha Yoga Pradipika*, written around 1350 CE by Swami Swatmarama. In this text are 15 postures, and 8 are seated postures.

A.J. Pollock

A.J. Pollock is a Major League Baseball player for the Arizona Diamondbacks. After being drafted in the first round out of the University of Notre Dame, he made his MLB debut in 2012. In 2015, A.J. was an MLB All-Star and won a Gold Glove Award. He ended his all-star season batting .315 with 20 home runs and 76 RBIs.

T.E. How did you get into yin yoga?

A.P. I have a lot of yang in my life, a lot of go, go, go. Right now, everything is geared toward how to maximize your recovery, especially in the sport I play. Everyone that I've given the yin DVD from your set *The Ultimate Yogi* to try out, the response has been just awesome. It's never like, "Yeah, I kind of like that." It's something like, "Wow! That's something that I really need!" For me, right away, it felt amazing. My sleep was way better. It was a meditation, but also a stretch where I got a lot of good stuff going on in my body. I really enjoy it and it's probably the number one thing I do on the road yoga-wise. I do it after games. It's huge the way I feel the next day. It's like a recharge for my whole body!

T.E. Have you seen an increase of yoga and meditation within baseball?

A.P. Definitely. Players who are looking for their peak performance, they're seeing that you need to have balance in how you train. I definitely see a willingness to go outside of what the traditional training is. Usually, it was old-school weight room stuff: Put the weight on your back and do squats or do the bench press. It's probably not as usable as yoga is when you get on the field. I think there's a big demand for yoga out there in baseball.

T.E. Can you describe some of the specific physical benefits of yin?

A.P. Well, first of all, when you're playing baseball, your legs feel awful the whole year! [laughter] Whenever there's a moment when you're like, "Wow!

My legs feel good," in baseball, it's not just, wow. "It's, wow! This is amazing!" This is like, "What's going on here?" [laughter] So yeah, I feel like there's a lot of blood flow. I feel like there's a big, warm sensation going on in my legs. It feels like my body is doing a flush, flushing inflammation out. I usually wake up feeling great. It helps with my range of motion. My body just feels more pliable the more I do it. I imagine it helps with injury prevention, and I definitely do it as a recovery.

T.E. How many time a week do you practice yin yoga?
A.P. I do it two or three times a week. The actual full hour that I want to do, maybe once a week. I'd say at least twice a week I'll be doing a version of yin yoga where maybe it's a half hour.

T.E. Do you have a favorite yin yoga pose?
A.P. At the moment, when I'm doing them, I don't like any of them! [laughter]

T.E. It's sort of a love–hate relationship. [laughter]
A.P. They're challenging. I like the one where we're falling forward, grabbing both legs, caterpillar pose. There's also dragon pose. That one gets into the groin, hamstrings, and the hip flexors. When we get to that one, as much as that one hurts, that one's excellent for me.

T.E. What about a least favorite yin yoga pose?
A.P. Fire log pose. I don't get it, and I've tried and tried. I'm not sure if my body is built to get my legs on the ground. I get through them and I do as much as I can. That one's a tough one for me, not exactly my strongest pose. [laughter]

T.E. Could you share any last inspiring thoughts?
A.P. Well, people ask how I got to the big leagues and why some other people haven't. I just say it's commitment. Just like anything in life, if you really want to be the best at something, then there's a huge commitment you have to have. Your actions have to follow that commitment. You never lose sight of what your ultimate goal is.

What some people overlook is how physical and athletic meditation actually is. If you've meditated for over 20 to 30 minutes, you begin to notice all sorts of sensations that arise within the body. You feel discomfort, aches, pains, and tension in the hips, knees, ankles, and spine. Sometimes the discomfort becomes so unbearable that you have to stop the meditation prematurely. The yogis, wanting to become fully liberated, used these postures to work out the kinks and make the body more supple. Then they could withstand longer and longer seated meditations. The yoga poses were created to support the meditation. This concept in the West has been lost by many.

In the late 1600s another hatha yoga text was released called the *Gheranda Samhita,* which expanded the posture library to 32 asanas. This particular text started to shift the game: Two-thirds of the poses were stronger with a yang-like quality, and just one-third had a softer, more yin-like quality. Up to this point, it had been the other way around. This trend continued as hatha yoga evolved into a more active, strong, and eventually athletic style. More yoga poses were developed, many of which were inspired by gymnastics, wrestling, and other exercise.

Krishnamacharya, known as the godfather of modern-day yoga, knew about 3,000 postures and taught vinyasa krama. This style of yoga links a movement with a breath and induces a powerful flow state. Krishnamacharya taught and inspired many legendary teachers, such as B.K.S. Iyengar, Pattabhi Jois, T.K.V. Desikachar, and Srivatsa Ramaswami.

Although it's beautiful on some level that yoga has become so popular and spread so rapidly, you can see how in certain ways it's become disconnected from its roots. If hatha yoga is about balance between the yang and yin, which we will dive much deeper into in the next chapter, and most classes are very yang-like, then we are creating imbalance.

When yoga began thousands of years ago, it was about meditation. And the earliest yogis meditated in a seated posture. They held this seated posture in stillness for extended periods, sometimes hours. As you will soon learn, this very much qualifies as **yin yoga**. From this perspective, the first form of physical yoga was yin yoga. It might not have had a name, but that's what it was. As we learned earlier, the seated poses of the Hatha yoga tradition became greatly diminished in favor of the strong standing postures. Like the element of water that yields eventually, the early forms of Hatha yoga adapted and, as yin yoga adapted, found a new and wonderful path that manifests even stronger and more transformative.

MODERN HISTORY OF YIN YOGA

In 2005, I signed up for a yin yoga workshop at Santa Monica Yoga. I had no idea what to expect or what I was getting into. From a little research, I knew that the teacher was a world-renowned kung fu artist and that he had developed this unique style of yoga. That's about all I knew.

The teacher came into the studio and I could tell just by the way he moved that he was a special breed. His movements were incredibly graceful as if he were gliding across water. His structure was slight, slender, wiry, and, for a highly trained kung fu artist, nonthreatening. If you happened across him a dark alley, you would not be scared at all. This is what they say about many of the great Taoist masters. These masters never stand out in a crowd. Almost magically, they are able to blend and disappear into their surrounding environment at will.

Over the next two to three hours, this teacher guided us through a series of movements unlike any yoga I had experienced before. It was primal and animal-like. The form was fluid. We moved all over the studio facing in all directions, and at times we held certain poses for extended periods. I could feel my muscles and joints opening in new ways. As the practice went on, the density of my body seemed to disappear. Heaviness transformed into lightness.

This teacher's ability to move through different poses was unparalleled. It was almost like watching a circus performer. In fact, I've never seen anybody enter and exit a full split the way he did. No human movement was out his domain. He was a total master of the human body and I was a fan! His range of movement and ability to control his body were jaw dropping.

The teacher was Paulie Zink. As legend has it, Paulie learned a style of martial arts called Monkey Kung Fu from his teacher Cho Chat Ling. Cho Chat Ling, originally from Hong Kong, was acquainted with a person who was sentenced to solitary confinement in prison for killing another man. While in jail and with nothing but time on his hands, this inmate studied the movements of the monkeys outside of his jail window. He incorporated these monkey movements with the martial arts he had learned as a child and a new form of kung fu was born. When he was released from prison, he began teaching Monkey Kung Fu to others. This discipline made its way to Cho Chat Ling, who mastered this special martial art and took it from China to California in the 1970s.

It is the responsibility of a teacher to pass his or her knowledge onto the next generation. So the time was right when Paulie Zink and Cho Chat Ling connected in California when Cho Chat Ling was looking for someone to pass the art form to. Paulie Zink had studied martial arts in his youth, so when he found Master Cho during his college years, he was the perfect person. For seven years, Paulie studied daily with his teacher. About four hours a day were devoted to strong (yang) martial arts training, and four hours were dedicated to the soft (yin) style of Taoist yoga. It was a perfectly balanced blend.

Eventually Cho Chat Ling had taught his student everything he knew. Once his duty was fulfilled, Master Cho returned to Asia, and as the story goes Master Cho never charged his disciple for the lessons.

Paulie Zink developed the art form into what he called Taoist yoga, a blend of martial arts and yoga. The yoga component emphasized long, deep stretches and had an internal focus. He taught his students to be aware equally of both the external and inner world. In 1989, Paul Grilley became a student of Paulie Zink. Paul Grilley wrote the following in his book, *Yin Yoga: Principles and Practice* (2012, xiii):

> *I contacted Paulie, and he graciously invited me to join his weekly class on Taoist Yoga. Paulie practiced poses for five to ten minutes at a time, chatting contentedly as he led the class. After nearly two hours of floor poses we would stand and do some moving yang forms that imitated the movements of animals. It was all very interesting and all very different from the hatha yoga I was teaching.*

> *I stopped training with Paulie after about a year. By then I understood the simple principles of yin yoga. I had practiced some of his yang forms and had even dabbled in some of his kicking and punching exercises, but my interests were the floor poses, and it seemed inappropriate to take up Paulie's time when he had several students who wished to learn all aspects of the Taoist Yoga he had to offer.*

> *When I started to teach long floor postures in my public classes the studio owners wanted to know what to name the style in their advertising. Even though I included many traditional hatha yoga postures in my classes, the long, slow holds were certainly different from what everyone else in the studio was teaching, so out of respect for Paulie Zink I suggested "Taoist Yoga." And that was the name I used for 10 years.*

Paul Grilley created an incredible yin yoga video. Viewing it was a pivotal moment in my life when I was healing my serious knee injury. His video provides multiple practices that have different emphases. He also includes educational lectures that explain some of the science related to yin yoga, inspired by anatomy teacher Dr. Gary Parker. Paul's other inspiration, Dr. Motoyama, who was a Shinto priest and held doctorates in philosophy and physiological psychology, was also an inspiration in introducing the concept of the chakras and the meridians.

So, you may be wondering where the name yin yoga came from when the original name was Taoist yoga. Enter yoga and meditation teacher Sarah Powers, of "Insight Yoga." Sarah Powers was led to Paul Grilley's yin yoga practice because of a back injury. In her book, *Insight Yoga* (2008), she writes the following:

My back injury inspired me to deepen my investigation of the less popular style of practice called Yin yoga with Paul Grilley. (Yin yoga is a system of long-held, passive floor poses that are similar to but not exactly like restorative postures.) Paul's style at that time was quiet and focused inward. He would come into a pose and we would all follow suit, remaining inward-focused, silent, and motionless until he moved to the next shape, the signal that we could as well. After a few months of this, I began to notice how my lower back seemed to be growing healthier and more comfortable each day. My active flow practice was continuing to develop a core stability in my ab-dominal and lower back muscles, while the Yin practice seemed to be stimulating the circulation of chi (life force energy) into my deep-est spinal region, helping regenerate the fluid content in the joints while increasing the health of my spine. I loved how I felt after each Yin session, which made me interested in learning more about how these long-held yoga postures influenced not only my flexibility, but my overall health and mental well-being. (p.8-9)

Sarah Powers studied yoga with Paul Grilley and went on to become an accomplished yoga teacher, instructing both strong and soft forms of yoga. She called the strong aspects of the practice the yang part and the soft aspects the yin part. Eventually, Paul Grilley fully adopted the name yin yoga inspired by his student Sarah. It was at this point that yin yoga became defined by this name.

The universe always has a plan. Things come full circle. Yoga, thousands of years ago, started as yin, and now, in modern times, it is emerging again as a significant style of yoga.

Govind Das

Govind Das is the owner and director of Bhakti Yoga Shala, an innovative bhakti-based yoga studio in Santa Monica, California. Govind Das and his family live overlooking the ocean in the Pacific Palisades. Govind Das leads bhakti yoga workshops and retreats and presents at festivals and conferences in the United States and abroad.

T.E. How did you discover yin yoga?

G.D. I discovered yin yoga in my own self-practice. Not always did I feel like doing a strong power yoga or vinyasa yoga practice. At times, my body would just really thirst for stillness in the yoga poses, so that's where I first started my own practice with yin. Then in 1999, I started to hear about this teacher named Paul Grilley, and I took a yin yoga workshop with him. I realized at that point that the things I had been doing actually had a name, form, and a structure to it. It was called yin yoga. Why I love the yin practice so much is because of its meditative and surrender-based way of practicing. It's a nonstimulating practice, in contrast to the yang-based practices, which are very stimulating, yin is completely the opposite. It's more soothing for the nervous system. Yin practice is about slowing down and really meeting yourself in the moment. It reaffirms the teachings of Ram Dass in *Be Here Now* and Eckhart Tolle in *The Power of Now*. There is nowhere to get to. It's a fabulous and a fascinating practice to dive into.

T.E. Is there anything you find challenging about yin yoga?

G.D. It can be incredibly challenging. [laughter] The most challenging thing is just being with yourself, especially when you've been in a pose for three, four, five, six, seven, eight minutes. You're feeling sensations that could be incredibly uncomfortable, or your mind is very loud and noisy. I feel like it is such a great life practice. It sets us up for being in relationships and especially in intimate relationships and partnerships. In these poses, what we're asked to do is just to sit with what is. We have to learn the incredible virtue of patience. There's a great saying from the Vedas about the one who has patience has the entire universe.

T.E. What is your favorite yin yoga pose?

G.D. I always seem to come back to the dragon pose. I love it because of its challenge, and I love it because it's a direct gateway into our hips. Our hips are our largest joint in our body. There are a few different variations we can play with to access different parts of our hips and hip flexors. But to close the eyes and to settle in for five minutes and to just watch the phenomena and matrix of all of these different aspects of ourselves just dancing with each other. I find it absolutely fascinating to watch the miracle of human life manifest and express itself and expose itself, all through a hip stretch. [laughter] Just a simple hip stretch.

T.E. Do you have a least favorite yin pose?

G.D. The one that maybe brings up the most, is the traditional yin-style child's pose, which is where the knees are together. The feet are together. It's a real tight and compact child's pose. I find when I'm in that pose, because it's so tight and compact, I find it very difficult to breathe. When I find it difficult to breathe, it can bring up a tremendous amount of anxiety and fear. On some level, it's a great practice because it forces me to slow down and really connect with the breath even that much more.

T.E. Do you have any last "yinspiration"?

G.D. There is a quote by Gandhi that relates to yin yoga; it is "In a gentle way, you can shake the world." Sometimes less is actually more. The practice of yin is so still and chill, and it's not fancy, but it's so powerful.

In this chapter we explored the history of yoga. As you can see, yoga is much more than postures. It is one of the oldest living traditions on the planet and is multifaceted. The various paths of yoga are like different trails up the same mountain. They may vary, but in the end, the destination is the same. For a yogi, the destination is to become fully illuminated and awakened. In our next phase of the journey, we will learn about another type of yogi, the Taoist. In the next chapter we will dive into the magical and powerful world of the Tao.

CHAPTER 2
ESSENCE OF THE TAO

"If a man hears the Tao in the morning and dies in the evening, his life has not been wasted."

—Confucius

In this chapter, we explore the mystical tradition of Taoism and how it relates to yin yoga. Taoism, like yoga, offers a powerful and insightful way of understanding our reality. We will learn about Taoism's roots and some of the key concepts of this ancient tradition, including chi, yin and yang, and the five elements of Chinese medicine and how these relate to the modern world. The goal of this chapter is to provide context for the inseparable relationship between yin and the Tao.

WHAT IS TAOISM?

Taoism is a philosophical path whose roots date back to around 550 BCE in China. **Tao** means the way or also a road, channel, or path. In early times, the Taoists were known as magicians and sorcerers who were able to perform superhuman feats. As legend has it, they were even able to conquer death and reach immortality. Taoists, ancient or modern, attune themselves to the great laws of nature, which extend beyond religion, gender, and nationality and apply to all of humanity. When we fight these laws of nature, we create our own suffering. When we align with these laws of nature, we tap into an invincible and indestructible power.

For thousands of years, ancient Chinese shamans devoted their lives to studying nature. Tribal leaders made offerings to the sky, earth, mountains, valleys, and rivers as a way to strengthen the connection between humanity and the sacred mystery. They believed that encoded within nature were the secret laws of the universe. Lifelong observation began to reveal certain patterns and rhythms that were then passed from generation to generation. The deeper the Taoists' focus, the deeper the revelations. Through various forms of Taoist practices, they began to tune into more subtle layers of reality, and they discovered that within all matter was an undercurrent of energy and vibration. One example of this is a Taoist meditation known as Holding the One. In this meditation, the practitioner starts by stilling the body and mind until thoughts, emotions and sensations cease. Once stillness is attained, then the 'mind of the Tao' is revealed. The mind of the Tao is consciousness that sees all things as one. On the surface, things appeared solid and concrete, but that was because their perspective was limited by what they could see and feel. Special practices like Holding the One took the Taoists beyond the limitations of the gross senses. As oneness was experienced, the Taoists practiced harmonious living with nature.

In 1905, Einstein theorized that the ultimate stuff of the universe is pure energy. For example, a table is typically made of wood. A closer examination of wood reveals that it is made of fibers. Now, what are fibers made of? They are made of patterns of cells. Going even deeper, it is revealed that cells are nothing but patterns of molecules. Under further investigation we discover that molecules are patterns of atoms which are made of subatomic particles. This includes electrons, protons, neutrons, and photons. According to particle physics, the world is fundamentally made of dancing energy; energy that is forever manifesting itself in and out of existence.

So, when the Taoists looked at a tree, they saw more than just the wood. Their enlightenment allowed them to see the tree as dancing energy. In his book, *The Dancing Wu Li Masters* (1979), Gary Zukov writes about the similarities between physics and mystical enlightenment:

> *A closer examination, however, reveals that physics and enlightenment are not so incongruous as we might think. Enlightenment entails casting off the bonds of concept ('veils of ignorance') in order to perceive directly the inexpressible nature of undifferentiated reality. 'Undifferentiated reality' is the same reality that we are part of now, and always have been a part of. The physical world, as it appears to the unenlightened, consists of many separate parts. These separate parts, however, are not really separate. According to mystics from around the world, each moment of enlightenment (grace/insight/ samadhi/satori) reveals that everything—all the separate parts of the universe—are manifestations of the same whole. There is only one reality, and it is whole and unified. It is one. (p. 270-271)*

Taoism recognizes both the inner and the outer world. Many people go through their entire lives without connecting inward. It's like somebody going through life looking down the entire time. All they see is the ground, grass, rocks, asphalt, bugs, and maybe some trash. They never look up. They don't know that right above them is the sky, clouds, birds, leaves of a tree, sun, moon, and stars. Can you imagine? They are seeing only half the picture. That limited perspective restricts their potential to experience what's truly possible.

> *"Form is emptiness and emptiness is form."*
> *—Prajna Paramita Sutra*

One who follows the Tao is interested in the entire picture. They move through the outer world while still connected to the inner world. They carve time out of their life to go inside. As the attention goes in, they begin to focus and concentrate. This focus penetrates the noise of thoughts into a substratum of deep quiet.

This concept of a world inside of you may seem strange and perhaps New Agey. I get it. Since the moment you were born, you have been bombarded with external stimulation. Much of this stimulation has pulled you away from what's happening internally. Through radio, TV, magazines, and billboards, you have been enticed to indulge in countless products by major corporations. They want you to buy their products and they spend millions of dollars to convince you that if you buy what they're selling then you will be happier. Of course, this is an illusion and it's also a potential trap.

Happiness comes from within you. When I say happiness, I'm not talking about a fleeting emotion. I'm talking about a deep state of happiness and peace that is unaffected by external factors. To reach this state, you have to look within. When you look within through the practice of meditation, contemplation, prayer, or practicing yin yoga, you find there is a world within. In this internal world are thoughts, feelings, memories, sensations, and emotions. The richness found there is worth more than money can buy. Everything you could ever want already exists within—all the knowledge, creativity, strength, inspiration, wisdom, and love is inside of you.

> *"The quieter the mind becomes, the more that you can hear." —Ram Dass*

By quieting the mind and finding the stillness of the inner world, the Taoist begins to experience a reality under the hardness of the muscles and concreteness of the bones, just as the ancient Chinese did in their solitary study of nature. On this deeper level is a river of energy. This subtle flow of energy exists anywhere and everywhere. It manifests out of space and then disappears into space, almost like the flicker of fireflies on a warm summer evening. Human life is like that firefly. One moment it is animated, and the next moment it is gone. Our human life arises out of its source, and then one day disappears back into its source.

As one Taoist master put it, the source of who we are is like a river of infinite oneness. Eventually, the river tumbles over a cliff and transforms into a waterfall. From far away, the waterfall looks like a big blanket made of a unified substance; a closer look reveals trillions of tiny drops of water falling toward the ground. Our human incarnation is like that drop of water—seemingly inseparable, flowing through space. Eventually the individual particles join together with all the other droplets of water.

WHAT IS CHI?

The Taoists call source energy **chi**. In modern Chinese the word chi means *breath* or *air*. However, the ancient definition encompasses much more than that. In fact, the concept of chi is so nuanced, it's next to impossible to translate it properly. Words like *life force*, *energy*, and *vital energies* get us closer to its meaning. In the yogic tradition, source energy is called **prana**. Both terms refer to the same thing; they just use different names.

Chi is the underlying energy that permeates all life, reality, nature, and existence. Chi powers the sun, which is the source of light that travels to earth and is absorbed by plants. The energy that we acquire from plants helps to fuel the human body. Chi is the source of all nature that governs the primary elements, which we will discuss later in this chapter. Chi sustains the rhythms of nature. When you walk outside on a brand new spring day and everything is fresh and alive, it is an expression of chi. When you see the flash of lightning and hear the crash of thunder, this is a manifestation of chi. It is the source of all forms of gravity and magnetism, helping to hold everything together in a state of balance. It is the gasoline in our cars, the electricity in our homes, the heat in our ovens. It is the fire in the digestive system, the movement of nerve impulses throughout the body, the source of our breath, the driving force for the sperm that reaches the egg. It is the spark of all life!

The Taoists dedicated much of their lives to harnessing the power of chi. They discovered that the more of this energy they could tap into, the greater the possibilities of human experience. One could be strong, vibrant, and radiant, transcending suffering and eventually reaching the supreme state of immortality.

From my point of view, I don't think they meant a literal state of immortality, although there is part of me that would like to believe it. They found a way to live in the spirit body, not just the human body. They knew that their purest essence was beyond destruction. From this place, they could transcend the very things that bind normal mortals. They transformed fear into courage, disease into health, conflict into peace, weakness into strength, ignorance into wisdom. A Taoist is an alchemist. Chi is the ingredient necessary for this transformation to take place.

WHAT ARE YIN AND YANG?

The Tao is the undivided oneness of the universe. From this Tao of oneness, chi gives birth to two opposing but complementary forces of energy known as **yin** and **yang**. Yin and yang are configurations of chi.

The school of yin-yang is attributed to a man named Tsou Yen. He is said to have lived in the early part of the third century BCE. Tsou Yen studied topics such as math, astrology, politics, and geography. Certain historians credit him with writing numerous essays on the concept of yin and yang, although these writings have been lost.

The literal translation of yin and yang are shade and light. This meaning comes from the Taoist describing the absence and presence of sunlight on a mountain slope. All things in the world of form and duality have a polar nature. Everything has an opposite: male and female, day and night, hot and cold, external and internal, positive and negative, and heaven and earth. Also, in a physical yoga practice, we have counterposes. For example, we might follow a backbend with a forward bend. We might follow a twist to the right with a twist to the left. So, part of our humanity is to move through this dance of constant change—with yin and yang. In our lives, we experience gain and loss, pleasure and pain, praise and blame, victory and defeat, life and death. This is the nature of the Tao.

While writing this book, I was honored to officiate a wedding for two very good friends. The groom is one my best friends from college who directed many of my yoga DVDs, including *The Ultimate Yogi*. His bride-to-be completed my 200-hour teacher training a few years back. I spent the week before their wedding crafting their ceremony, focusing on the theme of beginning a new adventure together. (On a side note, I was nervous and felt a tremendous amount of pressure. Despite being in front of people regularly to teach classes, I didn't want to mess up this important occasion. It was terrifying!)

On the wedding day, I was driving to pick up the groom from his hotel. I was also the best man, so I was doing double duty. On the way, I received a heartbreaking phone call: My father-in-law had just passed away. Although he had been dying gradually from pancreatic cancer, the news was still devastating. To make matters worse, my wife, Lauren, was out of the country teaching at a yoga conference in Norway. She couldn't get back for another two days. There she was in a tiny hotel room, all alone, dealing with the passing of her father.

Time stood still when I got the news. I felt overwhelmed. Here I was on my way to celebrate the genesis of a couple's new life together at the same time my father-in-law had just died. And this is the nature of the Tao. We all face gain and loss, joy and sorrow, and birth and death. The laws are inescapable.

> *"When you realize the truth that everything changes, and find your composure in it, there you find yourself in nirvana."* —Suzuki Roshi

Everything is in motion. Life is cyclical. It is the cycle of yin and yang that can never be separated. You can't have life without death. You can't go up without coming down. You can't be awake without sleeping. You can't have sweetness without the challenges. Yet for many of us, we strive to control. We cling to what we label as good. We try to avoid what we label as bad. This mentality imprisons us in a little box of misery. Inside of this box, we suffer because we are fighting the natural flow of the Tao.

I'd like to share with you a personal story of one of the biggest days of my life, when I found the Tao. On the first day of a yoga retreat I was attending, some of the other students and I went on a hike along the Na Pali Coast in Kauai, Hawaii. High up on the bluffs we could hear fierce waves crashing below, and we had the feeling that this had been the case since the dawn of time. The environment felt primal and powerful. We made our trek deep into nature, leaving all signs of civilization behind. As we descended from the towering cliffs toward sea level, we saw multiple warning signs along the trail: "Do not swim in the water." They even warned of the likelihood of death due to drowning.

When our group arrived at a beautiful cove filled with majestic waves and surrounded by jagged rocks, I ignored the warning signs and stripped off my shirt and swam out into the ocean. As I glided away from shore, an undertow grabbed me. It had a power and force unlike anything I had experienced before. I was snatched up by one wave after another and thrown down with backbreaking intensity. I was held under the surface far longer than I could hold my breath, and to my horror, I began to drown. The ocean current pulled me toward the razor-sharp rocks. I remember having the thought,

"Great, not only am I going to die, but I'm going to have my spine broken in the process." The little bit of hope that I had for survival was completely dashed. I was forced into a state of absolute surrender. Instead of fighting to live, I was now fighting to die gracefully. I was smashed on the rocks over and over until I blacked out.

When I eventually came to, I was drifting out to sea. After the events that had just unfolded, every muscle fiber in my body was beyond exhausted. There was no question, my time had come, and I didn't have the energy to fight for survival. I took one last breath and began to sink into the mystery that awaited. Fortunately, at that moment I was grabbed and rescued by Scott, another participant in the retreat. Scott had grown up as a lifeguard in the San Francisco Bay area and was waiting for me get away from the rocks. After a daring escape, he got both of us safely back to shore. Had it not been for Scott, I wouldn't be here writing this book.

Lying on the beach, I was very relieved to find that I hadn't been seriously injured despite the beating that I took. As we hiked back to the retreat center that afternoon, I couldn't help but see all the warning signs not to swim along the trail. The signs were everywhere, but I still had chosen to ignore them. Isn't this true in life too? It's like we get off course and the universe whispers in our ear, "Warning, don't go there." But, we don't listen and we continue. Then the wisdom of the Tao speaks more audibly, "I said, warning, don't go there." And of course, we still don't listen, so then the Tao screams, "You big fool, WARNING, DON'T GO THERE!" If we are lucky, we eventually get the message. If not, we pay the price. The wisdom of the Tao is always speaking to us. The question is, Are we listening?

"Nothing ever goes away until it teaches us what we need to learn." —Pema Chodron

I didn't listen and I paid the price. I almost paid the price with my life. In many ways, I had been fighting the natural flow of the Tao. This near-death experience taught me many things. It taught me to become an expert in surrender. I was forced to surrender to a power greater than myself. I was awakening from the small self to the big Self. It taught me that in the end, there is only love. In that moment of drowning, the only thing I thought about were the people who had loved me and the people I had loved.

The ocean washed away the things that were no longer serving me in a positive way. Our greatest challenges become our greatest blessings. I was walking down a new path, the path of Tao. The rest of the retreat became a celebration of life through yoga, meditation, chanting, good food, gratitude, and community. This was just the beginning. It was as if a door had been opened, and I had taken that first step into the other side. For the time being, one foot was in the old paradigm and the other foot was in this new world of finding the Tao.

Now, let's get back to yin and yang. We have seen the yin-yang symbol many times (see figure 2.1). This symbol is simple, yet quite profound. First, notice that the shape is a circle. This circle represents the ongoing flow of the Tao. It also represents the cycles that exist throughout all of nature. Second, you'll notice that the left side is predominantly light, which represents the yang energy. The right side is dark and represents the yin energy. Third, notice the S-shaped curve that runs through the middle. Instead of placing a straight line through the middle of the symbol, the Taoists wanted to convey the importance that yin and yang are never separate. The Tao is a constant dance between these polar energies. Each flows

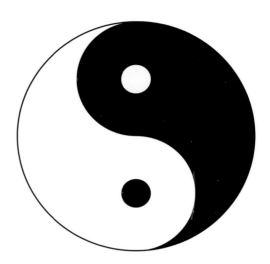

FIGURE 2.1 Yin-yang symbol.

seamlessly into another. Lastly, you'll see a small dark circle in the light part. There is also a light circle in the dark part. This shows that within yang, there will always be some yin. Conversely, within yin is some yang. Another key concept for yin and yang is that they are relative. I find it amazing that so much meaning is contained within such a simple-looking symbol.

Understanding the concept of yin and yang will provide the framework for seeing all perceptible things in a simple but powerful way. Yin and yang are aligned with subqualities that provide more texture to their meaning. The following list shows how each yin quality has a corresponding opposing yang quality.

Yin Qualities	*Yang Qualities*
Night	Day
Dark	Light
Cold	Warm
Negative	Positive
Passive	Active
Female	Male
Solid	Hollow
Stillness	Movement
Tranquility	Activity
Receptivity	Resistance
Moon	Sun
Midnight	Midday
Wetness	Dryness
Hidden	Revealed
Internal	External

We can also define people as exhibiting certain yin and yang features. Take a look at the following list and note which qualities apply to you. You might notice that you are a combination of the two. It's possible that you can have a yang body with a yin personality, or vice versa. Also, some of the qualities can shift from day to day. Although things are rarely black and white, these examples will give you another perspective on yin and yang.

Features of the Yin Person	*Features of the Yang Person*
Character: Quiet, withdrawn	Character: Assertive, aggressive
Build: Thin, small, soft	Build: Robust, muscular, tense
Energy: Slow, lethargic	Energy: Hyperactive
Posture: Limp, hunched over	Posture: Erect, rigid
Voice: Whisper, soft	Voice: Strong, loud
Body odor: Faint	Body odor: Strong
Breath: Light, shallow	Breath: Heavy, loud
Dislikes: Cold	Dislikes: Heat
Mucus: Clear, thin	Mucus: Colored, thick
Urine color: Clear, light colored	Urine: Dark
Stool: Light colored, loose	Stool: Dark, hard
Disease symptoms: Suffer intensely and recover quickly	Disease symptoms: Appear gradually and tend to linger

Although our culture tends to revere yang over yin, one is not better than the other. When yang is in excess, it depletes the life force and burns up the jing. **Jing**, in Chinese medicine, is considered to be the essence of human life. It is what fuels and nourishes the cells. The more jing we have, the greater length of life we have. Often, the yang personality lives hard and then dies hard. Someone who is a yang type can learn a lot from a yin type. They can find balance by slowing down, taking time to rest, practicing patience, and eating cool, nourishing foods. A yin personality can also learn a lot from a yang personality. They can adopt qualities that bring them out of their shell. Trying new things, taking risks, engaging in invigorating exercise, and eating warm foods can help bring them into greater balance. The key in Taoism is always balance and moderation. But as they say, "Do everything in moderation, even moderation!"

WHAT ARE THE FIVE ELEMENTS?

Tsou Yen, innovator of the school of yin-yang, is also credited with the teachings of wu-hsing, or the five-element theory. The five elements, as shown in figure 2.2, can be looked at as five phases that are related and connected to each other. They are the following:

Wood—Includes trees, vegetation, and minerals

Fire—Includes heat, light, sun, smoke, and fire

Earth—Includes soil, clay, rocks, and sand

Metal—Includes gold, silver, copper, and bronze; also, connected to magnetism and conductivity

Water—Includes liquid in the form of the oceans, rain, vapor, and moisture

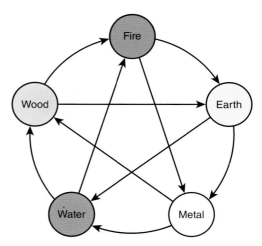

FIGURE 2.2   The five elements.

Understanding these five phases is important to being aware of the laws of nature. Each element, or phase, helps to produce or promote another. Each element is like a mother giving birth to another element. In another configuration of the five elements, they control each other through a promoting cycle and a controlling cycle.

Promoting Cycle

Water gives life to all vegetation, which promotes *wood*. Wood is the fuel and promoter of *fire*. After the fire consumes the wood, it creates ash, which promotes *earth*. Earth contains the minerals that promote *metal*. The minerals of metal become one and promote the element of *water*. The cycle is then repeated.

Controlling Cycle

Water puts out and controls *fire*. Fire melts and controls *metal*. The metal of an axe or chainsaw cuts down the tree, controlling *wood*. Wood and the roots of a tree dig into and conquer the element of *earth*. The earthen banks of a river control the flow of *water*. The cycle is then repeated.

The five elements provide a deeper perspective of the yin-yang model, and it's important to keep in mind that the two are always related. The number five was important to the Taoists. In addition to the five elements are the five seasons, five climates, five organ networks, and the five emotions. Chinese medicine is built on these concepts, and the subject could easily fill numerous books. For our journey into yin yoga, I hope to provide you greater context on the origins of yin. In our overactive yang culture, one of the most powerful ways to achieve balance is through yin yoga practice.

Almost a year after the near-drowning experience in Kauai, I signed up for a yoga retreat at Koh Lanta, Thailand. At the end of the retreat, I was invited to stay at the center to teach yoga. Honestly, teaching had never crossed my mind. I was happy just being a student. The prospect of teaching was exciting. I was also terrified. I had never participated in a yoga teacher training course, but yoga had become the love of my life. It was the thing that I was most passionate about. So, I said yes.

Those days teaching yoga and meditation on Koh Lanta were some of the happiest of my life. I was moving with the flow of the Tao. But the Tao is always in flux and changing, and I was about to receive one of the greatest lessons. This would be the lesson of impermanence.

One morning I was walking down the path toward my bungalow when I heard a voice screaming, "The water is coming, the water is coming! Get your stuff, the water is coming!" It was the Thai woman who owned the resort and she was in a state of hysteria. As I rounded the corner I could see that the ocean was surging inland. When I had arrived on Koh Lanta, the ocean had been blue and serene. Now, it was dark gray and ominous.

I ran to my beachfront bungalow and packed my stuff as quickly as possible. By the time I had lugged everything onto the patio, I was completely surrounded by ocean water. I was caught in a predicament. Do I abandon my things and swim to dry land? Or do I stay with my stuff and see what happens? After my near-drowning in Kauai, I wasn't too excited about getting into the water.

Then, the ocean water started to recede. It was like the plug had been pulled from a bathtub, and all the water was being sucked back out to sea. I was happy to no longer be surrounded by water. I found the highest hill I could, and I quickly dragged my belongings to what I hoped was a safe spot.

A few minutes later, as I watched from atop the hill, a wave three stories high came barreling down on top of our yoga retreat's restaurant. In the span of a few seconds, this entire structure disappeared without a trace. Soon after, a second wave followed, and like a boxer, the ocean delivered a powerful one-two knockout punch, destroying the beachfront resort.

I ran up to the main road and found utter mayhem. I jumped into the back of a crowded pickup truck. The driver sped us to the highest point on the island. When we got to the top, there were hundreds of people from all over the world and they were in shock.

We had been hit by a tsunami. It was December 26, 2004. A 9.0 magnitude earthquake, according to the U.S. Geological Survey, had released the energy of 23,000 atomic bombs. This gigantic force triggered killer waves that moved across the Indian Ocean at the speed of a jetliner. It was one of the largest natural disasters in recorded history and took approximately 250,000 lives.

High on top of that mountain, as the sun began to set, I made a pledge to the Tao. I would fully embrace its power and let it be my guide. I was committed to letting go of the small self, in order to embody the big Self. The human experience is fragile, especially in the face of nature. I had experienced this directly on two occasions. I was ready to dedicate my entire being to spreading the wisdom of the Tao through the teachings of yoga. The Tao is something, whether we know it or not, that is always moving through us. It is us. We are it. We are inseparable from the Tao.

They say that when you align yourself with the Tao, you no longer chase after things, they come chasing after you. It doesn't mean that the challenges go away and that everything is easy. You still have to keep showing up. You still have to keep being a student in order to learn and to grow. In a new way, you move through life with graciousness, purpose, and nobility. Anything not in alignment with that will fall to the wayside.

> *"The two most important days in your life are the day you are born and the day you find out why."*
> *—Mark Twain*

In this chapter we learned what Taoism is and where it comes from. We explored the intricate connection between nature and the Tao. The key concepts of chi, the yin-yang model, and the five elements provide a window of perspective into the way that Taoists view the universe. Most important, we devled into the context of the yin and how it relates to the yin yoga practice. Now that we've explored the essence of the Tao, let's continue to stay deep and journey through the subtle anatomy.

Stic

Stic (from the rap duo Dead Prez) is an internationally acclaimed hip-hop artist, songwriter, and producer who has come full circle as a passionate holistic health advocate. Stic is the founder of the RBG Fit Club, a lifestyle brand and website fusing hip-hop culture with holistic wellness. He lives in Atlanta, Georgia, with his wife, Afya, and their two sons, Itwela and Nkosua.

T.E. Can you explain, from your experience, what the Tao is?

S. It's been simplified as "It's the way." It's the unfolding of our nature in what and who we are. It's the understanding that there's a process that is ordered, even with chaos, that there is a flow and a wisdom to creation.

T.E. Could you could talk about chi?

S. I've learned in the teachings and in my experience that chi is everything. It's the vital life force, it's the evidence of the vitality in everything. It is also the evidence of function. So whatever is happening, it is the evidence of what is real, which is chi. So, the fact that we're breathing is evidence that there's a vital function that is happening, and the Chinese word for that phenomena is *chi*. In India, it's called *prana*, and in ancient Egypt, it was called *ra*. But, it's also important, I think to understand, that chi is not something that you're going to put in a jar and be able to quantify in a Western way.

T.E. What is your yin yoga practice like?

S. I do yin yoga on Tuesdays at 4:30 p.m. with my wife. It's a good supplement to running a lot. We are holding poses typically two minutes; sometimes we'll do five minutes for certain stuff. Again, it's the real power of being still and allowing the pose to do whatever it's doing. [laughter] I feel like it's about trusting.

T.E. What's your favorite yin yoga pose?

S. Well I'm going to have to say, it might be funny, but it's corpse pose. [laughter] Also, sleeping swan, just holding that and feeling that point of tension just relax at a certain point.

(continued)

T.E. Do you have a least favorite yin yoga pose?

S. I don't have anything that I'm like, "Oh, I hate doing this." But there's definitely lots of them that I'm challenged by! [laughter] You know what I've been having a challenge with? It's very simply just sitting and touching my toes, like the sitting forward fold [caterpillar pose]. My ego is like, "I want to be able to touch my toes easier," but I just haven't developed that flexibility yet.

T.E. Can you share any last "yinspiration"?

S. There's these two little rhymes that I like to be mindful of myself and share with the brothers because we get all "yanged" up. First is "Men need yin," and second is "Be strong, qigong." [laughter] Also, I have little Zen story that I really, really love.

It's about this farmer who lost his horse and his neighbor came over and said, "You've lost your horse, man, sorry about the bad news." And the farmer just says, "Who knows what's good or bad?" A couple of days later, that horse comes back, and it's followed by 13 other horses. In that time, if an animal is on your land, now you're the rightful owner. So, the neighbor sees all the horses and comes over to give him congratulations of good luck, and the farmer says, "Who knows what's good or bad?" A couple days later, the farmer's oldest son was riding one of the new horses and falls off and breaks his leg. And the neighbor, he's on top of everybody's business, he comes over and says, "Oh man, what luck, those damn horses! Your son broke his leg, that's messed up." And you know, the farmer remains calm and replies, "Who knows what's good or bad?" Sure enough, the king of the whole province wanted to expand his territory militarily, and he was drafting young men to go to war. And so, he stopped at the farmer's house looking for his oldest son. Of course, just so happened that his oldest son had a broken leg, so he didn't have to go to war. And you know, the moral of the story is, who knows what's good or bad? We have to let things unfold, stay centered, and attend to them as they happen without judgment.

CHAPTER 3
SUBTLE ANATOMY OF YOGA

"Everything in nature contains all the powers of nature. Everything is made of one hidden stuff."

—Ralph Waldo Emerson

Now that we have explored the essence of the Tao, we will dive into the subtle anatomy of the body from a yoga perspective. Subtle anatomy can be defined as a person's overall energy system that underlies the gross anatomy. When we address something as amazing and miraculous as the human body, we need to look at it holistically, as the Indian yogis and the Taoists did. By the end of this chapter you will have a greater understanding of what is taking place on a deeper energetic level.

FIVE KOSHAS

In yoga, our being consists of five **koshas**. Kosha can be translated as layers or sheaths. True health and well-being involves not only the physical body functioning effectively, but also all aspects of the subtle body doing so as well. According to the *Bhagavad Gita*, the subtle body is composed of the mind, intelligence, and ego and controls the physical body. As we learned in the last chapter, there is more to reality than what the five senses can detect. The koshas encompass everything from the superficial all the way to the purest essence of who we are. Misaligned koshas cause disharmony and fragmentation, leading to confusion and suffering. All the koshas must be united and blended if you are to achieve wholeness and illumination. The following are the five koshas:

Annamaya Kosha: Sheath of Food

This sheath consists of the gross anatomy of the body. It includes the skin, bones, muscles, and internal organs. It is called the sheath of food because nutrition provides the building blocks for these tissues. As they say, "You are what you eat."

Pranamaya Kosha: Sheath of Vital Energy

This sheath consists of breath, energy, and the chakras. This relates to what the Taoists call chi and the yogis call prana. We can increase the prana within our being by eating prana-rich foods like fresh vegetables and fruits. Spending time in nature and breathing in fresh, clean air, will also contribute to the health of this kosha. A regular pranayama practice will also keep the energetics of the body strong and vital.

Manomaya Kosha: Sheath of the Mind

This kosha has two layers: the mind and the heart. From a yoga perspective, these two are one and the same. The layer of the mind is related to our thoughts. The heart is related to the emotions. In yoga, we use meditation practices to direct our thoughts. The mind makes a great servant but a terrible master. For the mental state to be healthy, we must be in control of the mind. To have a healthy emotional heart, we must not hold onto toxic emotions such as anger and resentment. These negative emotions pollute this kosha. Forgiveness and loving-kindness meditation are powerful practices for keeping this kosha pure and healthy.

Vijnanamaya Kosha: Sheath of Causal Intellect
This kosha involves the higher self, the self where knowingness exists. We often look outside of ourselves for answers, but through the practice of looking within and quieting the mind, wisdom begins to emerge. This wisdom is innate to all human beings. This wisdom serves as a compass, guiding us across a sea of suffering to the island of true happiness. Time alone spent journaling, meditating, listening, and being receptive connect us to this kosha.

Anandamaya Kosha: Sheath of Pure Bliss
At the core of our being is our spirit that radiates pure bliss. This bliss is like a light that has the power to dispel all darkness, including fear, hate, and ignorance. It is a natural force that all humans are born with and doesn't have to be manufactured so much as it has to be uncovered. When the other koshas are pure, we can naturally feel and experience this bliss. Some people call it the God nature and others might call it original goodness. Often when we are in the presence of a saint or fully illumined person, their bliss nature can activate our bliss nature. This is the power of spending time around teachers and masters who help us to remember who we truly are.

It is important to understand that the koshas are not separate. They merge into one another like the colors of a rainbow. Moving through our lives with an awareness of these five koshas helps us to live in a deeper and more meaningful way. This understanding also helps to guide us through the world in a more holistic way. For example, if you go to the gym to exercise just to improve your physical experience, then you're affecting just 20 percent (1 out of 5 koshas) of who you are. At some point, you might start to feel that despite the visits to the gym, something is missing. In fact, if you go to the gym purely for vanity reasons and nothing else, it will only add to your suffering. To live to your fullest potential, you must strive to work within all the different layers of who you are.

PRANA VAYUS

In addition to the koshas, another important branch of subtle anatomy is the **prana vayus**. Prana, like chi, is life force and vital energy. It's what fuels all of life—from the energy that regulates our bodily systems to the energy that fuels the sun. It's yoga's goal to increase prana within ourselves so that we have more energy to fuel the things that are important to us. *Vayu* means wind or direction of energy. Prana vayus are the winds of vitality. Let's take a closer look.

Udana Vayu

This is energy that moves upward. Centered in the diaphragm, it moves through the lungs, bronchi, trachea, and throat and governs exhalation. Our oral expression is connected to udana in the sense that we communicate from what we feel in our gut and in our heart. If it is healthy, we experience joy, but if it is suppressed, we feel depression. Seal pose (p. 134) is a yin posture that stimulates udana as the chest and heart draw upward.

Apana Vayu

This is a downward flow of energy. It can be found in the lower abdominal region and pelvic cavity. We see apana manifested when making love and giving birth. Disorders related to apana include constipation, diarrhea, lower back pain, and sexual impairment. Squat pose (p. 110) is a yin posture that stimulates apana because the hips and torso drop toward the floor.

Vyana Vayu

This is the outward flow of energy that moves the life force from the core of the body into the extremities. It is associated with the circulation of blood and lymph and with the peripheral nervous system. Blocking this energy can cause circulation issues such as cold feet and hands. Corpse pose (p. 152) is a yin posture that activates vyana vayu as the arm and legs radiate out from the torso in all directions.

Samana Vayu

This is the inward flow of energy. It governs digestion, absorption, and assimilation of the food, liquid, and air that enter the body. Imbalanced samana may lead to loss of appetite, indigestion, and bloating. Caterpillar pose (p. 92) is a yin posture that activates samana as the torso and legs fold into each other.

Prana Vayu

This is the circulation of energy. Just as nature and the Tao flow in cycles, it is the nature of prana to flow circularly. Prana is connected to the breath, lungs, and diaphragm. It is responsible for inhalation, and an imbalance of prana vayu can cause heart palpitations, labored breathing, breathlessness, and asthma. Other symptoms of an imbalance in prana vayu are anxiety, fear, and nervousness. Seated diamond (p. 121) pose is a yin posture that supports prana vayu as the lower body forms an unbroken loop.

Not only do the prana vayus exist within yoga poses, but they also are demonstrated in nature. For example, let's explore the journey of the sun and how we perceive it here on planet earth. At dawn, even before we can see the sun, an expansion of light begins to spread across the sky. This is vyana vayu. Then right at sunrise we begin to see the sun rise above the horizon. This is udana vayu. The sun continues to rise until it reaches its zenith. Eventually, it descends and lowers beneath the horizon. This is apana vayu. After the sun disappears, light recedes and contracts. This is samana vayu. This cycle is repeated and the circle continues. This is prana vayu.

Understanding the prana vayus gives you a new way to look at the subtle energetics of the poses. Equipped with this knowledge, you can use a posture to cultivate balance when something feels off. For example, if you feel emotionally blocked or stuck, then you could do sphinx or seal pose as a way to lift (udana) and expand (vyana) your heart. If you've been giving to others all day (vyana), then you could practice child's pose or caterpillar pose as a way of bringing your energy inward (samana). The prana vayus are a powerful way of balancing your yin-yang energies.

THREE GUNAS

Throughout nature exist three primal forces that are manifestations of universal intelligence. They are called the **gunas**, or subtle qualities, and they underlie all of creation. The gunas represent certain archetypes within our mind—both on the surface and deep within our consciousness. We can also look at the gunas within different types of environments and even the food that we eat. The following are the three gunas:

Tamas
Characterized by inertia, stagnation, lack of movement, dullness, darkness, and heaviness, it is the energy that creates ignorance of the mind and stifles change and transformation. A classic example of a tamasic person is the couch potato. An environment that is polluted or oppressively hot or cold will have a tamasic quality. Heavy food, such as meats, processed foods, and food that lacks nutrients is tamasic.

Rajas
This is the energy of change, motion, activity, evolution, and growth. In the mind, it is the energy of desiring, wanting more, wanting to be successful, and wanting to be the best. When it is out of balance, rajasic people are overly competitive and inclined to sacrifice their integrity to get to the top, even if it causes pain and suffering. A type A personality is a prime example of rajas.

An environment containing a lot noise, traffic, activity, people, and stimulation has a rajasic quality. Spicy, sugary foods along with highly caffeinated beverages have a rajasic quality.

Sattva

Characterized by balance, harmony, stability, clarity, and lightness, a sattvic mind is happy, content, and awakened. The spiritual leaders in our community radiate sattva. We always feel good and at peace in their presence. Places in nature that are undisturbed by mankind are sattvic. This could be in the forest or the mountains or locations with various forms of water such as a stream, river, lake, waterfall, or warm, tropical beach. Fresh, natural, plant-based foods are sattvic in nature.

Health is maintained through a sattvic lifestyle and is usually impeded by rajas and tamas. Take the example of a person who chooses to go out partying regularly. Often alcohol is involved and possibly even drugs, which are both highly rajasic. Chances are the environment is stimulating and noisy, and the other people also demonstrate rajasic behavior. At some point, the rajasic partyers can no longer sustain themselves, and they become tamasic and go to sleep or even pass out. The next day, they wake up feeling exhausted and depleted. This is more tamas. Then they might go to brunch and choose to drink a few cups of coffee as a way to wake up and get going. This is more rajas. At some point, the caffeine wears off and they feel exhausted again and have gone back to being tamasic. The cycle simply repeats itself, until eventually the wisdom of the body steps in to shut everything down by getting sick. It's like an emergency off switch as the intelligence of the body tries to bring itself back to balance or sattva.

A vicious cycle of tamas and rajas is no way to live. It's like being on an out-of-control roller coaster, constantly shooting up and then falling down. Trust me, I know what this is like and I've been there before. It's difficult to maintain balance when it seems like the majority of people live this way, especially when we are younger.

Instead, you want to make choices that help reinforce the quality of sattva. Wise choices on where to go, what to eat, and who to surround yourself with will bring you more health and happiness. Even the things you watch, read, and listen to have an impact on your mental state.

Now with all that said, tamas and rajas aren't always negative. There is a positive way of looking at these qualities as well. At night, when it's time to go to bed, you need some tamas to fall asleep. Eventually, you fall into a deep, sattvic state of rest. When you wake up, a great way to start the day is with healthy rajasic movement and exercise that will create a state of sattva.

SEVEN CHAKRAS

The chakras are part of yogic subtle anatomy. In Sanskrit, **chakra** means wheel. Seven chakras run along the central axis of the spine in a channel called the sushumna nadi (see figure 3.1). Traditionally, the chakra system comes from tantric philosophy. In Tantra, the creation of the universe is understood through the dynamic interplay of Shiva and Shakti, similar to Yin and Yang in Taoism. The purpose of the tantric path is to realize that the world of duality is an illusion and that everything is one. The chakras are vortexes of energy that correlate to certain physical, mental, and emotional attributes along with an element, color and bija mantra. Bija means *seed*, so a bija mantra represents the essence of a chakra through the form of a sacred sound syllable. The chakras start at the base of the spine and run vertically all the way to the crown of the head.

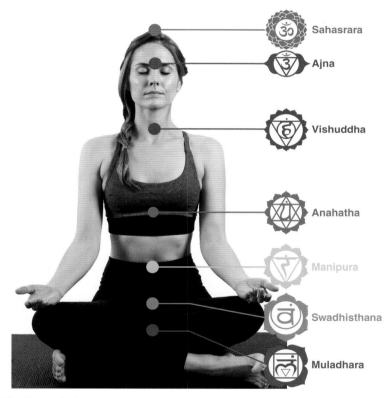

Sahasrara

Ajna

Vishuddha

Anahatha

Manipura

Swadhisthana

Muladhara

FIGURE 3.1 Seven chakras.

Muladhara

The first chakra is located at the base of the spine, and is therefore related to the feet, legs, and pelvic floor. Muladhara is connected to how we relate to the material world, to our financial, job, home, and food security. Without these basic needs taken care of, it's difficult to move along a spiritual path. So, it is the foundation for all the other chakras. This root chakra is connected to the earth element. Its color is red, and its bija mantra is *LAM*. When this chakra is balanced, we feel grounded, safe, and secure.

Swadhisthana

The second chakra is located in the region of the pelvic basin and sacrum. It relates to creativity, sexuality, and the reproductive organs. Swadhisthana is connected to the water element and therefore has a correlation to the moon. Just like the moon affects the tides, it also affects this second chakra. Its color is orange, and its bija mantra is *VAM*. When it is balanced, we have a healthy relationship with creativity, intimacy, and sex.

Manipura

The third chakra is located in the upper-abdominal, or solar plexus, region. It relates to our digestive system and is related to our gut intuition, confidence, and self-esteem. Manipura is connected to the element of fire. Its color is yellow, and its mantra is *RAM*. When it is balanced, we have a strong, positive role within society.

Anahata

The fourth chakra is located in the heart region. Anahata is sometimes translated as the unstruck sound. It relates to our emotional state, and yogis often refer to it as being the home of the soul. It is connected to the element of air, the color green, and the mantra *YAM*. When it is balanced, we have a greater capacity for love, compassion, and generosity.

Vishuddha

The fifth chakra is located in the throat region and is our vital communication center. Vishuddha is connected to the element of ether. Its color is blue, and it is connected to the mantra *HAM*. When it is balanced, we are able to freely express our feelings and truth in our relationships and the world.

Ajna

The sixth chakra is located at the third-eye area at the front of the brain. It is where we have the ability to transform through the use of intuition, dreams, visualization, and imagination. It is the seat of the witness that watches and observes the constant flow of reality. Like the fifth chakra, ajna, is also connected to the element of ether. Its color is purple and it is connected to the well-known mantra *OM*. When it is balanced, we are calm, centered, and connected to our higher guiding force.

Sahasrara

The seventh chakra is located at the crown of the head, the part that is soft when we are newborns. Sahasrara transcends all the elements, colors, and sounds. When it is balanced, we are connected to the source of all life.

Through the practice of yoga poses, chanting the bija mantras, and the use of visualizations techniques, we can cultivate balance throughout all seven chakras. Through these yoga practices, we awaken kundalini at the base of the spine in the muladhara. **Kundalini** is this primal energy. It is like a serpent form of prana or chi. Through the activation of the kundalini, we begin to awaken the higher chakras, and the goal is to merge the individual self with the cosmic self. This kundalini is incredibly strong, like a powerful voltage of electricity. If the body and nervous system are not properly prepared, then too much kundalini can blow the energetic circuits of the body. Therefore, it's important to practice slowly and steadily with a qualified teacher.

> *"Be humble for you are made of earth. Be noble for you are made of stars."* —Serbian Proverb

I've had the pleasure of visiting the beautiful island of Bali three times. Devotion is embedded within the Balinese culture: devotion to other people, to nature, and to the divine. Almost everywhere you go on the island, you see this devotion represented in the temples. They also build altars everywhere. If you pay attention, you'll see them behind homes, along the road, at street intersections, and at the entrances to stores and cafes. This devotion to nature supports the idea that the Balinese are woven of the same fabric as the Taoists.

My second trip to Bali was to colead a yoga retreat in the well-known town of Ubud. At one point, we heard about a local Balinese shaman who was said to be powerful and could do chakra readings. We invited him to visit us. He arrived with his translator, and both were wearing all white. Like many of the Balinese people, he had a calm and gentle demeanor.

After setting up, we sent in our first student. After about 15 minutes, we heard sobbing. After half an hour, the student came floating down the stairs looking as bright as a star! The afternoon unfolded like that for hours: a student went into the chakra session, sounds of crying came cascading down, and then the student appeared looking a decade younger.

I was the last to go. We started our session by doing a short meditation in which the shaman asked me to close my eyes and relax. After the meditation, the shaman held two L-shaped metal rods. He aimed the long part of the rods in the direction of the chakra so that they could do one of three things. They could swing away from each other in a sign that the chakra was open. They could stay parallel to each other, indicating that the chakra was neutral. Or the rods could cross each other, which was a sign that the chakra was closed.

If the chakra was closed, the shaman went into a meditative state to access information to determine why. He then brought up the challenging event that had caused the blocked chakra, which triggered an emotional release and healing. Then the shaman chanted to help purify the negativity from the chakra. He also prescribed a specific spiritual practice to sustain the strength of the chakra. Often this involved chanting the bija mantra while visualizing the color associated with its chakra. The work of the shaman was powerful because somehow he was able to intuit what was happening within the subtle anatomy.

After this experience with the shaman, I had a new respect and understanding of the chakras. This experience made them very real. Every person on that retreat felt the magic, mystery, and power of the chakra session. It was one of the peak experiences of the trip. The biggest highlight though, happened a couple of days later, and it was with the same shaman. He was about to show us what it really meant to be one with the Tao!

Sometimes you hear stories about Taoist or yogi masters who are able to levitate or walk through walls. Although I have yet to witness that firsthand, the following is a true story. A couple of days after our chakra reading with the shaman, we were invited to meet him again for a water blessing ceremony at a special temple. When we arrived, the shaman showed us around the grounds explaining what the various statues and buildings represented. Afterward, he asked everyone to sit in a semicircle, facing the front of the temple. He signaled that we would begin our water ceremony. He began ringing a bell and started chanting in an unfamiliar language. Although my brain had no idea what he was saying, a deeper part of me seemed to understand. Whatever it was, something was starting to stir. He continued chanting and ringing the bell. All of a sudden, the ringing and the chanting stopped. As the shaman looked slightly frustrated, he whispered to the translator. The translator stood up and adjusted our seated positions. It was like a world-class conductor fine-tuning the orchestra with great precision. The great symphony was about to begin.

The translator sat back down and the shaman picked up where he had left off. This time though, the intensity picked up. His chanting became louder, and the clanging of the bell became more ferocious. Suddenly, off in the distance, a cloud appeared. A big cluster of white moisture formed into a shape that hid the blue sky and sun. Just when I thought that the shaman could not become any more raucous, his energy surged, and the cloud danced its way across the sky in our direction. The closer it got, the darker it became. While the shaman was in complete rapture, the translator sat unmoving like a mountain.

By this point, we were on the verge of absolute rapture. The cloud positioned itself over our heads, and then the water blessing began. For about 10 minutes, rain poured down on our hot, thirsty bodies. Tears of disbelief soaked our cheeks. The group was shell shocked. With the shaman's power over nature, he was able to make it rain at will. It was a true gift and a blessing from the Tao.

Although for me this event was in the realm of miracles, the reality is that cultures dating back to prehistoric times have demonstrated power over the elements. Some call it magical Taoism. Someone who draws power from nature is considered a magician, whereas someone who draws power from spirits is considered a sorcerer. Taoist magicians are capable of manifesting rain, thunder, and snow, assuming they know the rituals and have cultivated enough personal power. My feeling is that our Balinese shaman was also connected to magical shamanism.

Regardless of whether we go on to become Taoist magicians ourselves, when we tune into our subtle anatomy, we can feel this part of us that's more than the confines of the physical body. Our real power resides in the subtle.

Before we wrap up this chapter, I would like to share with you a common saying from the people of Bali: "The people closest to God are babies and the elderly. The people furthest from God are middle-aged people with mortgages!" A little bit of humor is always good. As they say, never trust someone who is always serious!

In this chapter, we explored the subtle anatomy. Understanding these deeper layers of who we are helps us to see that human beings are complex and amazing and need to be examined holistically. Our yin yoga practice helps to awaken these deeper energies and therefore increase our potential as human beings. When the koshas are pure, the prana vayus flow freely, and the chakras are balanced, we are able to live a life of health, meaning, and purpose. Next, let's explore the science of yin.

Adam Griffin

Dr. Griffin is the founder and chief acupuncturist at Acutonix Acupuncture and Wellness Center. His clinics are a leading center for the practice of traditional Chinese medicine in the Los Angeles area. Dr. Griffin loves to cook for his family, backpack, fly-fish, and surf.

T.E. What is your take on the meridians?

A.G. When you look into a book and you look up meridians and you think about acupuncture lines as they traverse the body, what you're looking at is actually not Chinese medicine. The *Huangdi Neijing*, or *Yellow Emperor's Classic of Internal Medicine*, is the mother of all books. There are no meridians in the *Huangdi Neijing*. Much of what we know about Chinese medicine comes from this book. It's this huge encyclopedic text.

In the early 1900s, a French bank clerk named George Soulie de Morant came across a description of a word in the *Yellow Emperor's Classic of Internal Medicine* that he couldn't translate. It was called *mai*. He thought, "This looks like a nadi. I'm going to use this French word that would describe what we know about nadis. I'm going to call them meridians." But they weren't meridians. The word *mai*, thanks to other people being able properly translate this book, is a vessel. There's a big difference between a meridian and a vessel.

What if all of this idea of energy and meridians is a false translation or an improperly translated text? What if what we are really talking about is something like the vagus nerve? Maybe what we're talking about are things like the peripheral nervous system, central nervous system, nerve bundles, and blood vessels. The way acupuncture works is by stimulating blood flow to parts of the body, which hyperoxygenates areas of injury, which in my opinion, is really what yoga is. It's breath. What follows breath? Oxygen.

T.E. So you're saying that in order to stay true to the authenticity of true Chinese medicine, we need to reframe the word meridian to vessel?

A.G. Yeah, I think that the blood vessels, within the context of Chinese medicine, are the channels of the body. They are the way that the joints and the muscle tissue become nourished. They're the way the organs become nourished. In Chinese, they call this zang-fu. So really, acupuncture is about how can I increase or decrease circulation to a particular area of the body through the manipulation of these nodes, or acupuncture points, on the body. I can use a needle. I can use my hand. I can use herbs, and I can use chemicals within foods. I can use breathing techniques. I can use yin yoga poses.

T.E. Can you relate this to a yin yoga pose?

A.G. Let's talk about reclining butterfly pose. Here you are, lying on this mat and opening up your chest. You talk about the heart meridian, the pericardium meridian, but what you're really doing is opening up the lymphatic pathways. You are stretching all of these blood vessels across the chest. Deep breathing into the abdomen engages the vagus nerve, which opens up the parasympathetic nervous system, which allows your body to produce hormones, which allows you to heal.

T.E. How would you say Chinese medicine and yin yoga are related?

What we do within Chinese medicine and yoga, is really look at ways to expand the body's ability to move blood through the body. Oxygen cannot be separated from blood, so we're also talking about oxygen. Hormones cannot be removed from blood, so we're also talking about hormones. So, when you're talking about the blood vessels, what you're really talking about is the inherent structure of blood moving through the body to the heart, through the lungs, and away from the heart to the extremities. It's about how we can increase the flow of blood, how can we increase the flow of hormones and neurotransmitters through techniques like meditation, breath work, acupuncture, yoga, body therapy, and exercise. That's Chinese medicine.

CHAPTER 4

SCIENCE OF YIN YOGA

"The Church says: the body is sin.
Science says: the body is a machine.
Advertising says: the body is a business.
The Body says: I am a fiesta."

—Eduardo Galeano

In this chapter, we explore the science of yin yoga. When I first started practicing yin yoga, I knew that I felt better afterward, but I didn't know why. It wasn't until I studied Paul Grilley's *Yin Yoga* video that I started to understand the science behind what happens while holding a yin posture. Throughout my years as a yin yoga enthusiast, research was conducted into the intricacies of the human body. Now with endoscopic digital video photography, scientists continue to make discoveries about the cells and human body tissue. They can see things that had been hidden until now. Technology is affirming that there is no greater creation than the human body. Yin yoga has a powerful effect on our cells, tissues, nervous system, and other structures in the body. In this chapter we explore these effects, and it is my hope that the science will inspire your yin yoga practice even more as you find out what's happening deep under the surface.

ANATOMY BASICS OF YIN YOGA

To understand the bigger picture of anatomy and how it relates to yin yoga, we start with the basic structures of the human body. For many of you, this might be a review from your earlier education. If you were like me growing up, you may have snoozed through your biology, physiology, and anatomy classes. But it's important to grasp these basic concepts to fully appreciate the fascinating scope of yin.

Cells

We begin with the **cell**. All organisms are composed of cells, which in science are the building blocks of life. It is estimated that the adult human body contains approximately 50 trillion cells. All tissues in the body are built of cells, and most of the functions of physiology are performed within the cells. Although there are many remarkable similarities between cells, they also come in different shapes and sizes and have different functions. When you study cells under a microscope, they appear to be like little people. Instead of randomly bouncing around, they appear to function with purpose like a human being does. In fact, every cell that contains a nucleus (eukaryote) contains the functional match of a nervous system, excretory system, endocrine system, muscle and skeletal system, circulatory system, reproductive system, and even an immune system. Pretty wild, right? You are a collection of 50 trillion cellular "people." Then, in relationships, your 50 trillion little people cells interact with someone else's 50 trillion cells. No wonder relationships are so complicated!

The **cytoplasm** is the semifluid substance between the nuclear membrane and the cell membrane where the organelles (cell's organs) are located. Examples of organelles include the nucleus, mitochondria, endoplasmic reticulum, and the Golgi body. A scaffolding-like structure called the cytoskeleton gives the cell its shape and structure, along with holding the organelles in place. The **cytoskeleton** also aids in the cell's movement.

At the center of the cell is the **nucleus**. At the beginning of their life cycle, all cells have one nucleus, and this is where deoxyribonucleic acid (DNA) is found. DNA contains important genetic information. Conventional science adopts the belief that the nucleus is the cell's brain. However, a growing movement in science called new biology believes this might not be the case. Scientists have been able to extract the nucleus from a cell and prove it can survive for up to two months or more without genes (Lipton 2005). These enucleated cells are able to carry out complex behaviors, which demonstrates that the cell's brain must still be intact despite the removal of its nucleus. What the enucleated cells have lost are their reproductive abilities. As cell biologist Dr. Bruce Lipton states in his book *The Biology of Belief,* "...the nucleus is not the brain of the cell—the nucleus is the cell's gonad!" (2005, 42).

If the nucleus isn't the brain of the cell, then what is? According to Dr. Lipton, it is the **cell membrane**, or what he likes to call the "mem-Brain." This sheath that surrounds the cell and contains the cytoplasm is only seven-millionths of a millimeter thick. Some primitive microbes, called **prokaryotes**, consist of only a cell membrane and cytoplasm, yet are able to carry out the same functions as more complicated cells. Without a nucleus, they are able to eat, digest, breathe, eliminate, and survive. The cell membrane is the only organelle found in every living cell. Dr. Lipton describes the cell membrane as "a liquid crystal semiconductor with gates and channels" (2005, 72). So, what are the gates and channels? See figure 4.1 for an example of a cell and its parts.

The gates and channels embedded in the cell membrane are called **integral membrane proteins (IMPs)**. These IMPs are the key connection between the

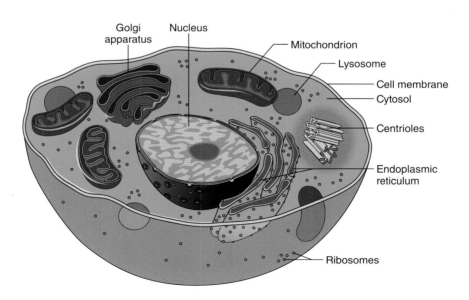

FIGURE 4.1 Parts of a cell.

individual cell and its surroundings. IMPs can be broken into two categories: receptor proteins and effector proteins. The receptors are like cellular antennas that monitor signals from the external environment. The effectors help to transport information from one side of the membrane to the other, synthesize molecules, and aid in the regulation of the shape and motility of cells. Simply put, one of the main functions of IMPs is to allow nutrients into the cell and eliminate waste out of the cell.

A certain type of IMPs are called **integrins**. Integrins link the cytoskeleton to the extracellular matrix. Through the integrins, important signals are expressed. The integrins act as a mediator or a two-way street. This is how the cell communicates to its external environment and how the external environment communicates to the individual cell. Without the integrins, there would be no cellular division, growth, or survival.

Although there has been extensive research on the cell, what about the environment that exists outside of it? It is so complex, that is has various names, such as **extracellular matrix (ECM)**, connective tissue, ground substance, and interstitial spaces. This extracellular world has been largely unexplored, but that is beginning to change. Researchers are finding a whole world within this part of the body.

Biophysicist James Oschman, PhD, calls this terrain the living matrix. Dr. Oschman is a leading researcher in the field of energy medicine and says, "The living matrix continuum includes all of the connective tissue and all of the cytoskeletons and cell nuclei throughout the body" (2016, 165).

> *"Don't look for miracles. You yourself are the miracle." —Henry Miller*

Connective Tissue

The most extensive structures in your body are **connective tissues**. These tissues connect, support, and bind body structures together. Without these connective tissues, the body would have no form and spill into a puddle of bones, organs, and muscles. The main functions of the connective tissue include providing support for the musculoskeletal system, protecting the organs, and assisting in the transport of key substances throughout the body.

Simply put, connective tissues build the substances that make the body strong and pliable, and they hold everything together. They bind the cells in the body together. The extracellular matrix is found everywhere from the skin all the way to the nucleus of the cell. It is the Tao of the body. It is through this vast network that the Tao of the body communicates, processes, and stores information. See how the dots are starting to connect?

Gray's Anatomy (1995, 80) defines the extracellular matrix as the following:

> *The term extracellular matrix (ECM) is applied to the sum total of extracellular substance within the connective tissue. Essentially it consists of a system of insoluble protein fibrils and soluble complexes composed of carbohydrate polymers linked to protein molecules (i.e., they are proteoglycans) which bind water. Mechanically, the ECM has evolved to distribute the stresses of movement and gravity while at the same time maintaining the shape of the different components of the body. It also provides the physio-chemical environment of the cells imbedded in it, forming a framework to which they adhere and on which they can move, maintaining an appropriate porous, hydrated, ionic milieu, through which metabolites and nutrients can diffuse freely.*

As you can see, the connective tissues are vast and complex. Their roles and functions are unparalleled. Included in the category of connective tissues are tendons, ligaments, bones, cartilage, joints, and fascia.

Tendons

A **tendon** is a tough band of dense, white, fibrous connective tissue that joins a muscle to a bone (see figure 4.2). Although different structures of the body are often depicted as separate in anatomy books, the reality is that there is a gradual continuum from muscle, to tendon, and then eventually into bone. Tendons function to transmit forces and withstand tension. Tendons are made of collagen fibers that ensure strength and flexibility and provide a natural resistance to being overstretched. A stretch of 4 percent is the limit of a tendon's flexibility. If the tendon experiences a larger stretch, the nervous system sends a warning signal to quickly relax the muscle. A stretch beyond this capacity could result in permanent damage to the tendon. The Achilles tendon, which connects the calf muscle to the heel bone, is a well-known example of a tendon.

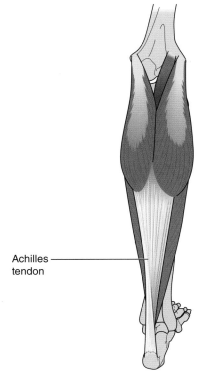

Achilles tendon

FIGURE 4.2 Tendon.

Ligaments

Ligaments are similar in constitution to tendons, but their function is to connect bone to bone, often supporting a joint (see figure 4.3). Generally, ligaments are darker in color and take various forms, including bands, chords, and sheets. Also made of collagen, ligaments are tough and incredibly strong and provide mechanical reinforcement and stability. One example of this is the anterior cruciate ligament which connects the femur to the tibia at the knee joint. Because of their high amounts of elastin, the most

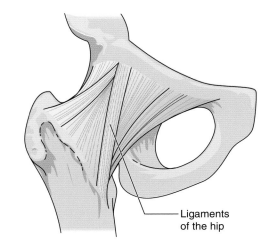

FIGURE 4.3   Ligament.

flexible ligaments are found in the lumbar spine and neck. It can be tempting to overarch these flexible areas, but it's important to avoid this. For example, in a yoga backbend, you never want to thrust your head back and overstretch the ligaments in the neck. Instead keep the chin positioned slightly down to ensure a long neck.

Bone

Bone tissue is a dense type of connective tissue that protects organs, produces red and white blood cells, stores minerals, and provides support and structure for the body (see figure 4.4). Osteoblasts are cells that build bone tissue. Often when we think of bones, we think of an image of a skeleton. These bones are often depicted as solid and a whitish color. These are cortical (compact) bones and are surrounded by a layer called the periosteum, which is composed of fibrous connective tissue. This fibrous connective tissue is made up of collagen that intertwines the periosteum and seamlessly connects with the ligaments and tendon. In flat bones, under the cortical bone tissue, is the trabecular tissue, which is the middle layer. This type of bone tissue is

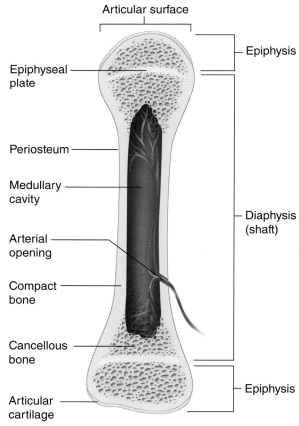

FIGURE 4.4   Bone.

lighter and spongy. Even deeper is the medullary cavity, which houses bone marrow. There are two types of bone marrow: yellow, which is made up of fat cells, and red, consisting of hematopoietic tissue, which is where the red blood cells, platelets, and white blood cells are made.

Cartilage

Cartilage is a firm but flexible tissue made predominantly of protein fibers (see figure 4.5). It is less complex than bone tissue, having fewer cells and minimal or no blood flow. It has a smooth, elastic quality. Two types of cartilage in the skeletal system are hyaline and fibrocartilage. Hyaline cartilage composes the septum of your nose and is the major component of the joints, especially synovial joints. In the fetus, hyaline cartilage helps in the construction of new bone. This bendy bone makes the baby a natural "yinster" in the

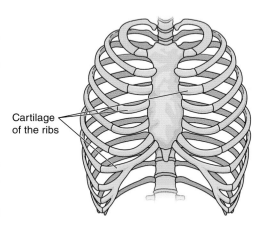

FIGURE 4.5 Cartilage.

womb. Fibrocartilage is a spongy tissue that serves as a shock absorber in the spine and pelvis. Cartilage protects the end of long bones at the joints. Chondrocytes are the cells that build new cartilage.

Joints

A **joint** is where two bones join together and link the skeletal system as a whole. Working in tandem with skeletal muscles, the function of the joints is to provide movement and bear weight in the body. The following are the three types of joints.

- *Fibrous*—Dense connective tissue that is rich in collagen fibers joins two bones in this type of joint (see figure 4.6*a*). These joints are also called fixed joints because they don't move. An example of this is where the radius and ulna bones meet in the lower arm.

- *Cartilaginous*—Cartilage joins two bones in this type of joint (see figure 4.6*b*). There is more movement in this type of joint than a fibrous joint, but less than synovial. An example of this are the discs in the spine.

- *Synovial*—A cavity exists between two bones in this type of joint. The cavity is filled with synovial fluid and dense connective tissue (see figure 4.6*c*). This type of joint produces the most movement.

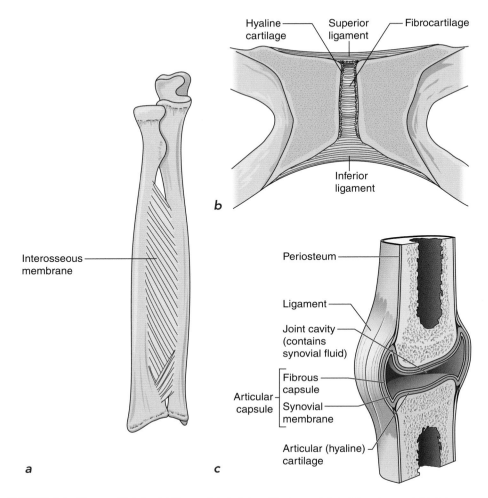

Hyaline cartilage

Superior ligament

Fibrocartilage

Inferior ligament

b

Interosseous membrane

Periosteum

Ligament

Joint cavity (contains synovial fluid)

Fibrous capsule

Articular capsule

Synovial membrane

Articular (hyaline) cartilage

a

c

FIGURE 4.6 Types of joints: *(a)* fibrous joint, *(b)* cartilaginous joint, *(c)* and synovial joint.

Fascia

Fascia is a type of connective tissue. Its name comes from the Latin word for band or bandage. One way to think of fascia is like plastic wrap or cling wrap for the body. It is an integrating tissue that envelopes the bones, muscles, and organs. Fascia helps to maintain posture, control body position, and produce smooth coordinated movement. The following are three types of fascia.

Superficial Fascia   The superficial fascia exists under the skin, or epidermis (see figure 4.7). The skin acts as a boundary between the outer and inner world. The next layer under the epidermis is the dermis. Although they are considered different layers, there is no separation between the two. Both of their

When Not to Yin

Yin yoga may not be appropriate for everyone. Someone with hypermobility is one example. Hypermobility, sometimes known as double-jointedness, describes joints that stretch farther than normal. Hypermobility is the opposite of limited range of motion. It is estimated that hypermobile joints occur in 15 percent to 20 percent of the population.

Hypermobility can be a result of the anatomical shape of ones bones or a connective tissue defect, such as Ehlers-Danlos syndrome, Loeys-Dietz syndrome, and Marfan syndrome. These conditions can create abnormal joint stress, causing the joints to wear out. These worn-out joints can lead to osteoarthritis. Hypermobile joints can be easily injured and contribute to muscle fatigue, chronic pain, and even permanent disability.

Hypermobile joints need to be stabilized. During movement, people with hypermobility must diligently activate the muscles around the joint. This typically involves the contraction and engagement of muscles to avoid collapsing into a joint. Because yin yoga's physical emphasis is on stretching the connective tissues, it can create problems for people who are hyper-flexible, but it also provides all the benefits of activating the parasympathetic nervous system (Birney 2016). What should this population do?

People with hypermobility, who don't need to stretch, have a couple of options when practicing yin yoga. They should do poses intelligently and use props to support the body. Learning how to do this requires studying with a knowledgeable teacher. The other option is to choose yin yoga's close relative, restorative yoga. As we explore in the chapter Developing a Personal Practice, restorative yoga also supports the body with props but, unlike yin yoga, the emphasis is never on looking for the edge of the stretch. A last option, when looking for a way to align with a yin energy on a mental level, is to develop a meditation or mindfulness practice. For more information on meditation refer to chapter 6, Pranayama and Meditation.

Another instance of when not to yin is during an acute injury. The two classifications of injury are chronic and acute. Chronic injuries develop slowly, take a long time to heal, and present mild symptoms. Acute injuries are the result of a sudden traumatic event such as a collision or fall and can occur while playing sports, while exercising, and during an accident. Common acute injuries are sprains and strains, torn ligaments, swelling, fractures, and dislocations. Symptoms of acute injuries include sudden, severe pain; swelling; inability to bear weight on the foot, ankle, knee, or leg; sudden loss of movement; severe weakness; and a bone visibly out of place. Someone with an acute injury should consult a doctor before starting a stretching program to ensure sufficient recovery has taken place. Keep in mind that as frustrating as injuries can be, they are also great teachers. They often teach us to slow down, be more caring, and to bring more yin energy into our lives.

movements flow in harmony. As we move deeper into the body, the next layer is the hypodermis, which contains the superficial fascia. The superficial fascia helps to maintain stability of form by providing the hypodermis with positive tension. Moving beyond the superficial fascia and hypodermis, the interfibrillar spaces are bigger and the fibers less rigid, and the tissues become more supple. This area is known as loose connective tissue, or areolar tissue. Loose connective tissue allows the tendons to slide smoothly. Where this tissue surrounds the

Fountain of Youth

Hydration within the deep fascia is important. The older we get, the dryer we become. This dryness contributes to joint stiffness and muscle tightness, which can accelerate the aging process.

Synovial fluid is secreted by the synovial membrane. This fluid is found within the synovial joints of the body, such as the elbow, knee, shoulder, and hips. This fluid has a thick, slippery consistency like an egg. Synovial fluid minimizes friction within the joint, making it easier for bones and cartilage to move past each other. This facilitates smooth and painless movement and serves as a natural shock absorber. When pressure is exerted on the synovial joint, the fluid becomes thicker to provide protection from the stress. When the stress goes away, the fluid returns to its normal viscosity. Another key role of synovial fluid is to supply oxygen and key nutrients. It also helps remove carbon dioxide and metabolic waste materials from the cartilage, where it is eliminated via the blood stream.

The body naturally produces the necessary amount of this lubricating fluid. I once heard that synovial fluid is like WD-40 for the body. If you've ever used WD-40, a spray lubricant, on an old bicycle chain or an old door hinge, then you know how it can work wonders. Maintaining the correct amounts of synovial fluid within the body will produce a type of "slide and glide" effect.

Hyaluronic acid (HA) is a type of ground substance and has been described as nature's moisturizer. The ground substance is the fluid that fills the space between the fibers and cells of the bodily tissues. This fluid is made up of a variety of proteins, water, and glycosaminoglycans (GAGs). Water makes up approximately 70 percent of the ground substance. What attracts the water are the GAGs, and one of the most important GAGs is HA.

HA, a crucial component of the extracellular matrix, is created by fibroblasts. This gelatinous substance can be found in almost every cell of the body. It occurs in greater concentrations in the bones, cartilage, tendons, ligaments, and other connective tissue. It has been estimated that HA can attract and tendons is known as the peritendon. In addition to helping aid the movement of tendons, loose connective tissue also helps to activate muscle contraction.

Deep Fascia   The deep fascia is the structure that is most pertinent to yin yoga. It is located under the subcutaneous tissue (see figure 4.7). This tissue is much thicker and tougher, composed mostly of tightly woven fibers. It envelops and penetrates the muscles, bones, nerves, and blood vessels. Deep

contain one thousand times its volume of water. This attraction of water helps the body tissues stay hydrated, lubricated, and springlike. The hyaluronic acid separates, supports, and cushions the living cells within the connective tissue. This cushioning allows the connective tissue to endure the tension, pressure, and stress that no other body tissue can.

HA, along with other GAGs, play an important role within the synovial fluid to ensure that the joints work properly. As mentioned earlier, the synovial fluid brings in nutrients and removes waste. HA facilitate this. Hyaluronic acid is found in large amounts in the lips, eyes, gums, and the skin. In fact, roughly 50 percent of HA in the body is located in the skin. HA, along with collagen, helps to maintain the skin's structure so it remains smooth and elastic. The moisture that HA provides gives skin its youthful appearance. HA has a lifespan of about three days. To remain healthy, it is crucial that the body replenish HA. This becomes more challenging as we grow older because the fibroblasts that create HA diminish as we age. As the HA decreases, the skin can no longer retain moisture. At this stage, skin becomes dry, rough, and wrinkled (Clark 2012).

This is true of the connective tissues as well. They too can become dehydrated, stiff, and less elastic. The extracellular matrix becomes filled with more fibers. As this occurs, the fibers stick to each other, creating adhesions that decrease mobility, and circulation suffers, resulting in decreased flexibility and increased fatigue and bodily pain. To make matters worse, toxins and waste products get stuck where the adhesions take place, and harmful bacteria can multiply rapidly in these areas. Cellular communication becomes impaired, and the toxins create abnormal electromagnetic impulses that are disruptive to the natural intelligence of the body. This limits the ability of the cells and tissues to function optimally.

Although aging is a natural process, we have the ability to slow the process through the continued production of HA. Yin yoga stimulates the production of hyaluronic acid through deep stretches of connective tissues. This is why yin yoga is commonly referred to as the fountain of youth.

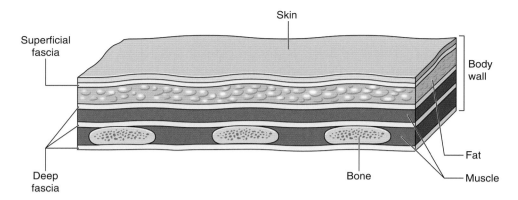

FIGURE 4.7   Superficial and deep fascia.

fascia is made up of collagen, which provides tissue strength, and elastin, which provides tissue resiliency.

- *Collagen*: The word **collagen** means glue producer, and it originally referred to the boiling of animal parts to obtain glue. Collagen has incredible strength and is the main component of fascia, cartilage, ligaments, tendons, bone, and skin. It keeps the skin strong, strengthens blood vessels, and helps to build tissue by facilitating the role of fibroblasts.

- *Elastin*: **Elastin** is a highly elastic protein found in the connective tissue. After tissues in the body are stretched or contracted, elastin returns the tissues to their original shape. Imagine if you pinched your skin and pulled it away from the body and then when you let go, your skin was left drooping from the body. (Not a pretty sight.) Fortunately, elastin in the body keeps this from happening.

The deep fascia serves many important functions. Within the deep fascia are an abundance of sensory receptors that detect pain, changes in movement, fluctuation in temperature, changes in vibration and pressure, and changes in chemistry. Based on this sensory input, the deep fascia adapts by contracting, relaxing, or shifting its compositional materials. For example, in the event of a sudden emergency, the body shifts into the fight or flight response, which induces strong contractions within the fascia. This rapid contraction can give normal people Herculean strength. When you hear stories about mothers able to lift cars to save their children, this is why they are able to. Bolstered with tensioned fascia, people can tap into extraordinary levels of strength.

A **fibroblast** is a type of cell that builds collagen and is the most common type of cell in the connective tissue of animals. The primary function of fibroblasts is to maintain the structural integrity of connective tissues by secreting materials that create the extracellular matrix. In addition to providing key structural support, they also play a pivotal role when tissue has been injured. They act as an emergency responder, alerting the immune system to invading microorganisms and setting the stage for recovery to begin.

The collagen and certain proteins in the extracellular matrix make the fascia stronger and thicker. Collagen is often referred to as a "complex protein" because it contains 19 amino acids. Glycine is one particular amino acid found in collagen that produces muscle growth. Although this produces more strength within the body, it can come at a price. In some circumstances, the body begins to lose its suppleness, and wherever the buildup of extra collagen has taken place, range of motion suffers. A classic example of this is professional bodybuilders. Although they have massive muscles, they are unable to move the body in all the ways it is capable of moving. For bodybuilders simple tasks such as taking off their shirts, tying shoes, or scratching their backs become nearly impossible. In this case, strength has actually become a hindrance (Clark 2012).

What's the point of having strength if you can't use it? The good news is that the extracellular matrix can restore flexibility when the contractions relax. By relaxing the fascial system, a remodeling of sorts takes place. The extra material that was created through the sustained contraction is eaten up by macrophages within the extracellular matrix. Macrophages are a type of white blood cell that eat up cellular debris, foreign substances and cancer cells; they are like the janitors of the cellular world. The components of the fascial material will then produce more elastin and restore the tissues' flexibility (Clark 2012).

Subserous Fascia   Although yin yoga doesn't directly affect this third classification of fascia, I want to discuss it so that you are informed. Think of this as a little extra credit. The subserous fascia, sometimes called the visceral fascia, supports and suspends the organs within their respective cavities (see figure 4.9). Each organ is wrapped in dual layers of fascia that are separated by a thin serous membrane. If these connective tissues are too loose (yin), then it causes organ prolapse (displacement of an organ), and if they are too tense (yang), it restricts optimal organ function. Even on this very deep level of the body, we see the importance of balancing yin and yang.

Science of a Yin Pose

You have probably heard the expression "No pain, no gain." Typically, this applies to a workout situation. The idea is that if you don't exercise to the point of pain, then you are wasting your time. Some people hear this and then they go out and hurt themselves. This is a tricky expression because it depends on the situation. The reality is that there is good pain and there is bad pain. Bad pain is when bone is grinding into bone or too much physical stress is exerted on a particular body part. Usually, in this kind of situation, the pain will manifest as a sharp sensation, burning, or numbness. This is your body's way of telling you that the situation is negative. On the other side of the coin is good pain. For example, when you get a massage from your favorite massage therapist and they dig their elbow into a knot of tension in your back, it's painful. It doesn't feel good in the moment. As they work out the kink and get blood circulating through the area, the tension releases. Then you start to feel better. You find comfort after moving through discomfort. In contrast, if a therapist is overly aggressive in their touch or digs their elbow into a bone, such as your spine, bad pain will be triggered and your body will revolt.

Similarly, when you work within a yin yoga pose, it's important to be able to tell the difference. You want to imagine that you are both the giver and receiver of the massage. Exposing areas in the body that are stiff, atrophied, and tight will create uncomfortable sensations, but that is the good pain you are looking for. Good pain is another way of saying positive stress. In yin yoga, you want to work with this concept of positive stress.

To initiate the healing effects of yin, you exert positive stress on the tissues. The three types of stress are compression, tension, and shearing. Compression presses tissues together. An example is holding a rubber stress ball in your hand and squeezing, or compressing, it. Tension stretches the tissue; think about a rubber band or a piece of salt water taffy and how you can stretch it. Shearing is another way of saying twisting. Wringing out a sponge is a good example of shearing.

In our yoga practice, we perform all three of these actions on our tissues. Just like you can purify a sponge of its accumulated toxins by squeezing, stretching, and twisting, so too can you do that for the body. In fact, yogis believe that the human body is like a big sponge that absorbs whatever exists within its environment. Unfortunately, pollution is a real problem in many parts of the world and those toxins end up in the body's tissues. Wringing out the body daily is one of the best things you can do to stay healthy and help the body rid itself of toxins.

Now let's connect the dots by imagining that we are doing a yin posture, the sleeping swan pose (see figure 4.8). Your front leg is bent, and your back leg extends straight behind you. The torso folds over the front leg. Depending on your body, you may have support under your front hip or a block under the forehead. As you come into the posture, the first thing is to *find your edge,* the wall of resistance that keeps you from proceeding farther, and gently lean into it. You know that for yin, time is on your side, so there is no rush to get anywhere. With the mind quiet, listen to any biofeedback being communicated through the language of bodily sensation. Fine-tune the pose, looking for your sweet spot. You are like a musician searching for the perfect pitch. As you find your perfect pitch, find stillness with a gentle movement of breath waving in and out through the nose. Initially, as you come into the pose, you will stretch key muscles such as the hip flexors, psoas, piriformis, and the erector spinae. You are exerting a positive stress on these muscle tissues.

In other styles of yoga, you might come out of the stretch after 30 seconds, but this limits the benefits that happen when you allow time to flow. After about 90 seconds is a

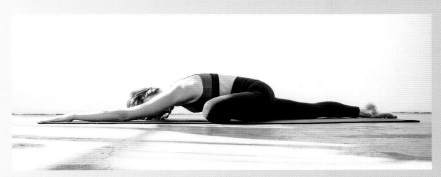

FIGURE 4.8 Sleeping swan pose.

phase change, where you begin to access the deep fascia and connective tissues, such as tendons, ligaments, joint capsule, and even the bone. This is when you start to reap the benefits of the good stress. By pressurizing the exposed tissues, you create a positive stress effect. At this point, the fibroblasts go to work. As you stress the fibers within the fascia, the fibroblasts secrete chemicals that rearrange the collagen, making the tissues stronger. The fibroblasts provide a similar function within the rearrangement of the elastin fibers, making the fascia more supple. This process has a positive effect on the tendons and ligaments because you are stressing them in a yin manner too.

In this sleeping swan example, the key structures that benefit are the hip and iliotibial band. This fibrous band runs along the outer thigh and is said to be so strong that it can support the weight of a car. How they figured that out, though, I don't know! Because of the spinal flexion, sleeping swan also stretches the ligaments in the lumbar spine. Typically, the ligaments in the lower back are the most flexible in the body. As you get older, though, the elastin fibers become mineralized, cross-linked with other fibers, and therefore more restricted. However, holding this type of deep stretch keeps the elastin fibers cleanly organized, and the ligaments remain healthy.

In addition to positive effects on connective tissue, yin yoga benefits the bones as well. Earlier we learned that the outer covering of the bone, the periosteum, is made of fibrous connective tissue. If the periosteum is unhealthy, bones will snap like a dry tree branch under pressure. However, exerting positive pressure on the bones stimulates the body's fibroblasts to increase the collagen of the periosteum. As more collagen is created, the periosteum adapts to the pressure by becoming more durable and resilient, like a living tree. Over time, it's as if you are exerting pressure on the branch of a living tree instead of a dry, dead tree branch. Because a living tree is hydrated and flexible, this elastic nature makes its branches much more difficult to break.

This is why when you practice, you often feel it in your bones. You actually move that deep into the body when you practice yin yoga. The entire fascial matrix is pressurized and benefits. After three to five minutes, you slowly exit the sleeping swan. Commonly, you feel tenderness within the stretched areas because it takes a long time for the connective tissues to open and also takes a long time for them to revert to their original positions. That dull, achy sensation you feel is a good sign. Because the connective tissues are connected into a vast network, the benefits of your yin practice will benefit every movement that you do. You'll most likely notice that it improves your sleep quality too by releasing unnecessary tension.

Spine

The spine, according to yogis, is the most important channel in the body. It is the foundation of your entire physical existence. The majority of the nourishment that your brain receives comes from the movement of the spine. You can live without an arm or a leg, but you can't live without your spine.

The spine starts at the skull and extends down to the pelvis. Ligaments in both the front and back run the length of the spinal column. The spine is made up of 33 bones, including 24 vertebrae and the fused bones of the sacrum and coccyx (see figure 4.9).

The following are the regions of the vertebral column:

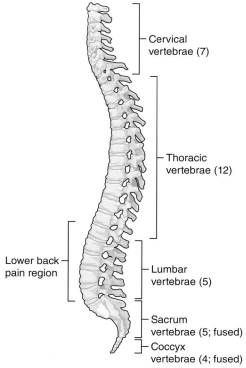

FIGURE 4.9 The spine.

Cervical

The cervical region of the spine contains seven vertebrae in the neck. The skull attaches to the top of the cervical spine via the atlas. The atlas comes from the Greek story about Atlas, who held the world on his shoulders.

Thoracic

The thoracic region is the middle of the spine and contains 12 vertebrae. The ribs attach in this area.

Lumbar

The lumbar region of the spine contains five vertebrae in the lower back. This area takes the most stress, especially in modern-day living due to excessive sitting while working, driving, and eating.

Sacral

The sacral region of the spine contains five vertebrae fused into the sacrum. This area connects the hip bones and last lumbar vertebra.

Coccygeal

The coccygeal region of the spine contains four vertebrae fused into the coccyx, or tailbone. This area protects the overall spine from the shock of sitting.

Located between each of the vertebrae is an intervertebral disc, which is made of fibrocartilage. This and the natural curves of the spine provide shock absorption. When you look at a healthy spine from the side, you see that it curves four times: forward at the neck (cervical spine), backward at the chest (thoracic spine), forward at the (low back) lumbar spine, and then backward at the hip area (sacral spine). The forward shape is known as a lordotic curve. The backward shape is known as a kyphotic curve. In addition to protecting the spine from shock, the spinal curves also aid in balance, and they position the head over the pelvis, which enables you to walk upright.

The spinal column protects the spinal cord, which is part of the central nervous system. The spinal cord is the superhighway that the brain uses to send messages throughout the rest of the body. It is composed of white and gray matter. The white matter is nerves that are covered with myelin. Myelin, made of fat and protein, is a fatty white substance that insulates the axon of some nerve cells. Gray matter lacks myelin covering, making its appearance gray in color instead of white. Essentially white and gray matter are large bundles of nerves that carry information via the spinal cord. These nerves are connected directly or indirectly through other nerve branches related to the spinal cord.

Dr. Jeremy Brook, known as the Spine Checker, is a chiropractor and anatomy teacher in Los Angeles, California. He says the following about the spine (2009, 17-20):

> It is nature's most powerful and intricate architectural masterpiece. The spine is built for protection and stability, flexibility, locomotion, respiration, and for achieving super-conscious states of being. We have to take extreme care of this important instrument. This is because the spine is at the core of everything. Everything is suspended to the spine. It is the infrastructure of the body. Unfortunately, we now spend an average of sixteen hours a day in a seated position, without proper preparation and in chairs. Sitting is to the spine what hard candy is to the teeth! The average American has lost the S-curve in the spine and in many cases has a reversal of the curve in the neck. Every day, all day, I see people who have lost their natural curves in the neck. The spine was built to protect the spinal cord and to act as the core infra-structure for our life! Sitting puts pressure on the nervous system and interferes with the body's ability to communicate with itself and maintain balance and vitality. With a loss of curve, weight distribution is removed from the joints and placed upon the discs. Our spinal discs dehydrate, flatten, lacerate and herniate, setting up loss of function and increased pain and suffering. So now you're asking yourself . . . what can I do? An easy proactive step along with chiropractic care is to commit yourself to a yoga practice. The body is built for movement!

As you can see, the spine plays a pivotal role in our health and well-being. If this is the case, then why is it often neglected in many forms of exercise and fitness? It probably has something to do with the fact that it's not a vanity body part. You'll see people in the gym strengthening their chest and bicep muscles and toning their glutes, but you don't normally see people doing exercises solely for their spinal well-being. Fortunately, the Taoists and the

Yin Yoga and Pregnancy

Although yin yoga is a therapeutic activity for most, a small part of the population should proceed with caution. One of these groups is women moving through pregnancy. I have had the pleasure of being indirectly involved with the act of giving birth as the father of two beautiful kids: Lantana and Bodhi. I watched their mother navigate through all the ups and downs of pregnancy and use yin yoga to help facilitate the process.

Moving through a yin yoga practice with awareness can create a state of calmness and serenity. When a pregnant woman feels serene, her confidence is stronger. When she is serene, her stress about the process of childbirth can be minimized. Practice allows her to become present by attuning to the natural sensations of the body. Intimacy, compassion, and love are strengthened. It is beautiful that these same qualities can shift from pregnancy into motherhood.

Before starting a pre- or postnatal yin yoga program, it is important to obtain your physician's consent. Approach your practice while pregnant with sensitivity, respect, tenderness, and care. During pregnancy, the body is changing, the blood chemistry is shifting, and the miracle of life is growing inside of you. Probably more than anything, the quiet mindfulness that yin yoga practice provides is much needed. Keep in mind that the body's chemistry changes with a greater release of **relaxin**. This increases flexibility in the ligaments and can lead to overstretching. This, along with other important information, is listed in table 4.1.

yogis did, and as we continue to explore, you will see how remarkable yin yoga can be for you and your spine.

Now, please don't think that I'm disparaging people who go to the gym. I'm a big fan of cross-training. I'm just advocating for making choices dominated by your wisdom over your vanity.

"A flexible spine is a flexible mind." —Yogi Bhajan

TABLE 4.1   Yoga Practice Tips for Pregnancy

First trimester (weeks 1-13)	This is the time when morning sickness can cause symptoms of nausea, dizziness, and tiredness. Avoid practicing during these episodes of sickness. • Avoid all twisting poses, even modified twists. • Lying on the belly is OK, but breasts are often sore. • Lying on the back is good, especially because you can't in the second and third trimester. • Don't hold your breath; it worsens dizziness. • Inversions like legs up the wall and supported bridge are OK.
Second trimester (weeks 14-28)	The baby bump is starting to show. • Avoid lying on the back and the belly. • Avoid all deep backbends. • Energy in the body returns. • The hormone relaxin increases in the body, which relaxes pelvic ligaments. • The baby doubles in size. • The second trimester presents the highest likelihood of injury to the mother, so practice with extra sensitivity. • Listening to intuition is important.
Third trimester (weeks 29-40)	Avoid lying on your back. • Risk factors for baby have decreased, but always proceed with care. • This is the time to mentally prepare for childbirth. • Take big breaths with audible exhalations. • Drink plenty of healthy fluids to avoid dehydration.
Postnatal (post birth for 40 days)	Mom creates the energetic environment for the baby. It is best for mother to sleep when the baby sleeps to enhance recovery. • Be patient, some women's recovery takes a year. • Relaxin will continue to flow through the body as long as you are nursing. • Work to repair the pelvic floor through exercises that involve adduction of the inner thighs. • Rebuild the core muscles by strengthening the transverse abdominis, the deep muscle that runs along the front and side of the abdomen. • Regain full function of your body through a strong and slow practice that concentrates on contracting the muscles to support the joints.

Desi Bartlett

Desi Bartlett, MS, CPT, E-RYT, is a leading pre- and postnatal yoga expert. Desi holds advanced certifications in yoga, personal training, pre- and postnatal fitness, and group fitness. She has worked with several celebrity moms in Los Angeles.

T.E. In what ways are a yin yoga practice beneficial during the various stages of pregnancy?

D.B. We all carry yin and yang energy: feminine and masculine. Masculine energy drives; it is all about action. Feminine energy receives. Yin yoga allows us to receive a sense of calm. The longer holds can also lead to a greater feeling of release in the hips and lower back. It is important for the pregnant mama to make sure that she does not try to achieve her deepest stretch in any pose, as the ligaments are a bit lax with the spike of relaxin. However, she can go into a comfortable stretch and then meditate on all that she is receiving: a deeper breath to share with her baby, a sense of calm in body and mind, and being birthed as a mother.

T.E. What positions and activities should a pregnant woman avoid in her yin yoga practice?

D.B. It is contraindicated to lie flat on your back or on your right side for extended periods of time during pregnancy. Lying flat or on the right side can put pressure on the vena cava [the large vein carrying blood to the heart], thus acting like a rock on a water hose; it compromises the flow. It is important for the mom-to-be to modify her yin practice so as to lift her head above her heart, or in poses like legs up the wall, have a bolster under her low back, with the tailbone able to drape over the front of the bolster.

Additionally, deep twists and prone positions (lying on your belly) are contraindicated and must be modified to accommodate the woman's changing body and to make space for the baby inside. It is important to remember that the spikes in relaxin will make the woman's joints a bit less stable, and it is important to not go to the deepest point of any stretch as she might not be able to feel the natural edge of the stretch.

Lastly, if the mom-to-be has been diagnosed with PJSD [pubic joint symphysis disorder], she cannot safely go into poses in which the legs are wide open. If she has been having SI [sacroiliac] joint pain, it is important to work with a skilled yoga teacher to make sure that the pelvis is well aligned in several poses, so as not to exacerbate the pain.

T.E. What advice and tips do you have for postnatal yin yoga?

D.B. New moms can greatly benefit from a yin practice. The body has been through so many dramatic changes and it needs time to integrate these changes. When women return to vigorous exercise too soon, it can cause some problematic situations in the harmony of the inner unit—meaning that the pelvic floor, transversus abdominis, diaphragm, and multifidus may see an imbalance in the system and not work together in harmony because one muscle group is stronger than another.

Enjoying a yin practice can also inspire a feeling of calm, which will help her body to counteract the stress of being a new mom. Motherhood is a joyous event, but even good stress is interpreted by the body as stress and can lead to a fight-or-flight response in her nervous system. The deep breathing and long holds hallmarked in a yin practice act as a salve for her nervous system. The opposite of fight or flight is called recovery and repair, and that is exactly what her system needs at this time.

T.E. Anything else that you think would be good to share?

D.B. Pregnancy is an amazing time in a woman's life. The only "should," is to listen to your body and honor the feedback. If the body needs to take it easy, a yin practice can feel amazing. Practices like yin yoga have been referred to as a "work in" (vs. a workout), as they can bring a sense of support and balance to our inner body. Yin allows moms to enjoy the sense of receiving, and that is a hallmark of this time in her life as she gets ready to receive her baby into her arms and into her life.

My hope is that after you have read this overview of human anatomy, you have an understanding of the physical effects of practicing yin yoga. If you would like to dive even deeper, know that entire books are dedicated purely to the topic of fascia. See the bibliography for some suggestions. But what you should understand at a minimum is that throughout the body is connective tissue that unites the various parts of the body and performs sophisticated functions. What happens in one area of the body ripples through the entire body. If this network of connective tissue becomes unhealthy, then the entire system suffers.

Good Pain Versus Bad Pain

As a yoga practitioner, it is important to be able to discern the difference between good pain and bad pain. Part of the human experience is to feel natural discomfort within the body. Inevitably, in your yin yoga practice you will be in positions where you encounter difficult sensations, and this is quite normal. If you have been to a massage therapist, then you understand what good pain is. They frequently take their thumb or elbow and dig into knots of tension within your body. While this is happening, it doesn't feel all that good, and you might even notice a grimace on your face. But what happens after they finish working out the knot of tension? Chances are, you feel tremendous relief. Hopefully, the massage therapist also brought a certain level of sensitivity to the process. Even though they were digging into the muscle tissue, there should have been a quality of respect. When this happens, you will most likely return to that therapist for further treatment.

Your yin yoga practice, in a way, is like getting a massage. The main difference is that you are both the giver and the receiver of the massage. This means that if you are attuned to your body, then you should be able to find that perfect spot of discomfort that is beneficial without being too much.

How do you know whether it is bad pain? Feeling sharpness, numbness, or a burning sensation is your body's way of telling you that something is wrong. In this case, you have a few options. First, you can try backing out of the pose. Sometimes you have just gone too deep too fast, and the body isn't ready for that depth. Second, you might want to explore one of the modifications offered in the pose descriptions. Sometimes using a prop for support can help immediately. Any time the body loses anatomical integrity, the law of compensation kicks in. In the event of misalignment, other areas of the body are forced to compensate, and usually this strains these areas. Last, sometimes because of the way your body is built, some positions will never feel right. It doesn't matter how much stretching you do, the pose won't improve. In this case, find a variation that exposes the same muscle groups but is more suitable for your body.

Bone grinding into bone is never a good sign. Always look for the stretch within the deep fascia. It is common when coming out of a long yin pose to feel tenderness and sometimes a dull, achy sensation. Never rush yourself within the transitions. Allow your body the time that it needs to adjust to the deep stretch that it just experienced. Bring mindfulness into each and every movement.

YIN AND YANG
OF THE NERVOUS SYSTEM

The human nervous system is evolution's way of creating a method for the mind to communicate with its 50 trillion cells. Its function is to perceive the outer world through the senses and then to broadcast that information to every cell through its integral membrane proteins. This enables all of your cells to work as a collective community. This harmony among cells, tissues, and organs increases efficiency and productivity and is a key to survival.

What Is the Autonomic Nervous System?

The human body is designed to seek balance. In science, this is known as homeostasis. The **autonomic nervous system**, which regulates the functions of the body, is one of the many ways that we see homeostasis in action.

I vividly remember eating at a cafe one afternoon when my daughter was a toddler. Her mom had ordered sushi. On the side of the plate was a small mound of green stuff. My daughter, who loved avocado, exclaimed, "Yummy. Guacamole!" Before we could stop her, she had shoveled a huge spoonful of wasabi into her mouth and swallowed. In about two seconds, her faced flushed bright red, her eyes rolled demonically into the back of her head, her mouth flew open, and then she vomited all over the table. Just another day in the life of parenting a toddler, right? The body is amazing, and when something isn't right it knows how to self-correct. Had she not expelled the wasabi, she could have done serious damage to her G.I. tract.

The system in the body that plays the biggest role in homeostasis and regulation is the autonomic nervous system. The autonomic nervous system, sometimes called the subconscious nervous system, is important to maintaining health. It controls heart activity, blood pressure, breathing, intestinal activity, temperature regulation, and multiple other functions, all automatically, without you having to make it happen. It's easy to take these functions for granted, but they are definitely something to feel grateful for. I like to look at this automatic intelligence as another manifestation of the Tao. The autonomic nervous system consists of two connected parts: the sympathetic nervous system and the parasympathetic nervous system.

Sympathetic Nervous System

The **sympathetic nervous system** is responsible for energy production and the body's ability to adapt to stress. It is typically more active during the day. Some of the ways that it interacts with the body is by dilating the pupils, inhibiting the flow of saliva, accelerating the heartbeat, dilating the lungs, slowing digestion, producing adrenaline and glucose, and inhibiting bladder contraction.

The sympathetic nervous system is related to what is commonly known as fight or flight. Travel back in time and imagine that you are a caveman or cavewoman out on a mission looking for food. Suddenly, you see a powerful beast charging from out of the bushes at you. It is a ferocious saber-toothed tiger and it thinks you are its next meal! In reaction to the tiger, your stress response is unleashed. The hypothalamic–pituitary–adrenal axis, called the HPA axis, springs into action. A tidal wave of cortisol, adrenaline, and other stress hormones from the adrenal glands flood through the body, causing you to either fight the tiger or run away from the tiger. Assuming you survive like your ancestors did, after the stressor (the tiger) is gone, your stress hormones normalize, and all is fine.

Flashing to the present, the saber-toothed tiger has been replaced by a different type of stressor. This stressor is modern-day life and includes traffic, the news, bills, deadlines, family commitments, climate change, and politicians constantly instilling fear about the latest threat. Maybe just reading that last sentence causes a stress response. Sorry about that! Unfortunately, that list isn't exhaustive, and much more could be added. One way our present-day scenario is different from that of our ancestors is that we can't run away from our stressors. We are swimming in a stress-overloaded reality. Many people are stuck in a chronic state of stress and sympathetic nervous system activity.

There is no greater enemy to your health than stress. Stress, more than anything else, presents the biggest potential to wreak havoc in every aspect of your life: your health, relationships, job, school studies, physical performance, and overall capacity to enjoy life. Potential sources of stress may include the following:

- *Physical*—Causes include poor dietary choices, allergens, physical trauma, overexertion, physical inactivity, illness, and lack of deep sleep.
- *Emotional*—Causes include relationship breakups, death, illness of a loved one, unresolved anger from the past, and suppressed emotions.
- *Social*—Causes include political situations; loss of a job; financial issues; and unhealthy relationships with coworkers, family members, and people in your community.
- *Environmental*—Causes include exposure to environmental toxins, computers, cell phones, household appliances, and fluorescent lights.
- *Spiritual*—Causes include a lack of purpose, lack of connection to a higher power, lack of faith, and being disconnected from nature.

Stress elevates the stress hormone, cortisol. Anytime your stress level skyrockets, your cortisol level also goes through the roof. Here are some of the effects of chronic, elevated cortisol levels.

Increased food cravings	Increased anxiety
Fat gain	Panic attacks
Shrinking of the brain	Increased depression
Immune system suppression	Mood swings
Diminished sex drive	Decreased brain function
Decreased muscle mass	Increased PMS symptoms
Decreased bone density	

A 2007 study published in the *Journal of the American Medical Association* states, "Exposures to chronic stress are considered the most toxic because they are most likely to result in long-term or permanent changes in the emotional, physiological, behavioral responses that influence susceptibility to and the course of disease" (Cohen, Janicki-Deverts, and Miller 2007, 1685). The damaging results of stress also affects one of the most important organs in the body, the brain. Stress is highly damaging to the brain because it causes the brain to degenerate and shrink (Kharrazian 2013).

Negative stress is a major risk factor for heart disease, cancer, gastrointestinal disorders, skin problems, neurological and emotional disorders, the common cold, arthritis, herpes, AIDS, Alzheimer's, and dementia. Sleep disorders are also linked to stress. To benefit from healthy sleep there must be a normal cycle of hormone production, especially cortisol. When things are properly balanced, your cortisol levels should be highest in the morning (6-8 a.m.) and lowest in the evening. As you fall asleep, cortisol levels should decline, and then the body releases the sleep-enhancing hormones melatonin and serotonin, providing a deep, recharging sleep.

However, for millions of people, stress interferes with this process. When we are overwhelmed with stress, cortisol levels remain elevated late into the night. This prevents deep, restful sleep. When this problem persists, the cycle of cortisol production can turn itself upside down, causing a major imbalance. In this case, cortisol levels are low in the morning, causing you to feel depleted and exhausted. Often, when people are exhausted, they develop an addiction to caffeine to give them energy. However, this is a false energy, and the caffeine exacerbates the imbalanced cortisol cycle. During proper, restful sleep, your cells remove toxins and repair themselves. It doesn't take much to put two and two together. If you are not sleeping properly, you are decreasing cellular health and greatly increasing the risk of disease.

In short, the more stress you have in your life, the more dominant the sympathetic nervous system is; therefore,

- the more your sleep quality will suffer,
- the more tired and fatigued you will be,
- the more inflammation will harm your cells, tissues, and organs,
- the more accelerated the aging process will be,
- the more you will experience negative emotions,
- the more likely you will be to experience restricted cognitive function, and
- the more likely you will be to become sick and suffer from major illness.

Keep in mind that although there is bad stress, there is also good stress. Certain types of stress are an important part of staying healthy, and your body is dependent on good stress. Earlier in this chapter, we explored putting positive stress on the connective tissues to make them stronger and more durable. An example of this lack of positive stress on the body is what happens to astronauts in outer space. Without the positive stress of gravity on the body, they experience loss of muscles mass and bone density. The factor that determines whether stress is negative or positive is whether the body perceives the stressor as a threat. If it does perceive it as negative, the body shifts into defensive mode. In summary, negative stress refers to any factor that causes physical, mental, or emotional tension that disrupts the body's equilibrium. It is the precursor to disease.

The following list summarizes the functions and emotions related to the sympathetic nervous system.

Functions	*Emotions*
Protects the body against attack	Will
Associated with fight or flight	Anger
Elevates blood pressure and blood sugar	Desire
Increases body heat	Fear
Regulates the brain, muscles, thyroid, adrenal glands, insulin, cortisol, and thyroid hormones	Irritability
	Guilt
	Depression

Parasympathetic Nervous System

The **parasympathetic nervous system**, in contrast to the sympathetic nervous system, is responsible for energy recovery, regeneration, repair, and relaxation. It is usually more active at nighttime. Some of the ways that it interacts with the body are to stimulate the flow of saliva, slow the heartbeat, constrict the lungs, stimulate digestion, stimulate the release of bile, and contract the bladder. Generally speaking, the sympathetic nervous system is related to performance, and the parasympathetic nervous system is related to rest and recovery.

> *"When you have a strong parasympathetic nervous system, you are going down stream."*
> *—Dr. Michael Galitzer*

The stronger your parasympathetic nervous system, the healthier you will be. Any coach of a world-class athlete will tell you that the body becomes stronger in a state of rest, not activity.

Cutting-edge doctors are speaking about the importance of healthy parasympathetic activity. Dr. Michael Galitzer and Larry Trivieri, both nationally recognized experts in integrative medicine, state the following (2016, 64):

> *The parasympathetic system is devoted to nourishing, healing and rebuilding the body. When actively dominant, it stimulates and enhances immune function, circulation, digestion and overall gastrointestinal function. It improves functioning of the liver, stomach, pancreas and intestines. It also lowers heart rate and blood pressure levels, while increasing production of endorphins, your body's "feel good" hormones . . . Only when your body is in a state of parasympathetic dominance are you able to achieve deep levels of rest and recuperation. Achieving and maintaining a healthy parasympathetic state is essential for healing on both the physical and mental-emotional levels of your being. Parasympathetic dominance enables you to be more relaxed, content and fully present in the moment. You are able to meet and respond to daily life challenges both calmly and more energetically.*

The parasympathetic nervous system is closely related to the vagus nerve, which is the primary pathway that the parasympathetic uses to send nerve impulses and signals. The vagus nerve originates in a part of the brain stem called the medulla oblongata. From here, it travels all the way to the colon, providing parasympathetic nerve fibers to the organs along the way. Because of this, the vagus nerve helps to regulate the homeostasis for a majority of the body's internal organs and the functions they perform. This includes heart rate, respiration, and gastrointestinal peristalsis. It is also involved with vision, hearing, speech, and control of the skeletal muscles.

The more rest and restoration you experience, the more dominant the parasympathetic nervous system, and therefore

- the more you can effectively manage stress,
- the better your sleep quality will be,
- the more you will be able to regulate the body's inflammation response,
- the healthier the cells will be,
- the better you will feel,
- the higher your brain performance will be,
- the more you will slow the aging process,
- the healthier and happier you will be, and
- the higher your quality of life will be.

The following list summarizes the functions and emotions related to the parasympathetic nervous system.

Functions

Heals, regenerates, and replenishes the body

Aids rest and recovery

Activates assimilation and elimination

Improves immune function

Regulates liver, kidneys, pancreas, spleen, stomach, small intestine and colon, parathyroid hormone and bile, and pancreatic and digestive enzymes

Emotions

Contentment

Gratitude

Serenity

Calmness

Relaxation

Enhancers

Eating potassium-rich foods (e.g., avocado, bananas, dark leafy greens) and using potassium supplements

Consuming warm drinks and avoiding cold drinks or drinks that have been sweetened

Drinking peppermint, lavender, and linden (tilia) teas

Performing deep-breathing exercises

Gargling

Singing loudly

Practicing yoga (of course!)

Meditating

Yin and Yang of the Autonomic Nervous System

To be healthy, we have to find balance within the human body. The sympathetic nervous system is connected to the energy of yang, and the parasympathetic nervous system is connected to the energy of yin. When this balance is lost, we can suffer from autonomic nervous system dysfunction. In their book, *A New Calm*, the authors Dr. Galitzer and Larry Trivieri Jr. write the following (2016, 44-45):

Autonomic nervous system dysfunction, or dysautonomia, nega-tively affects the nerves that carry information from the brain and spinal cord to the heart, bladder, intestines, sweat glands, pupils, blood vessels and especially the vagus nerve. There is a wide range of health concerns created by autonomic dysfunction, which might include excessive fatigue and thirst, excessively high or low blood pressure, irregular heart rates, difficulties breathing or swallowing, constipation and other gastrointestinal problems, bladder and uri-nary problems, and sexual problems such as erectile dysfunction in men or vaginal dryness and orgasm difficulties in women. Autonomic dysfunction also can be a factor in chronic fatigue syndrome, fibro-myalgia, irritable bowel syndrome and interstitial cystitis.

That is quite a list, and unfortunately, it gets worse. Dr. Galitzer and many other doctors are discovering new research on how sympathetic dominance is emerging as a primary cause of the biggest killer diseases on the planet, like heart disease, cancer, and stroke.

Dr. G. Blake Holloway is a neuroscientist and clinical naturopath and has an education in functional biology, clinical nutrition, orthomolecular medicine, applied psychobiology, behavioral science, biophysics, addictionology, and acupuncture. He is also the creator of NuCalm, the only patented system for balancing and maintaining the health of the autonomic nervous system. Dr. Holloway states the following about the sympathetic nervous system (quoted in Galitzer and Trivieri 2016, 86):

People who suffer from addiction and/or PTSD (post-traumatic stress syndrome), and also those for whom anxiety and depression are a problem, are essentially stuck in sympathetic nervous system domi-nance.

We know that the traditional model of treating PTSD by prescribing phar-maceutical drugs is failing because of the high suicide rates, especially among returning veterans. In the current model, those who benefit the most are the drug companies. In fact, Dr. Galitzer and Larry Trivieri write the following in their book *Outstanding Health* (2015, 340-341):

The ongoing use of pharmaceutical drugs is one the primary causes of dementia and other brain conditions, including delirium, in the elderly. This is especially true of people who have been prescribed more than one drug at a time. Common side effects related to the brain that can be caused by regular drug use also include anxiety, "brain fog," depression, erratic behavior patterns, and suicidal thoughts. In certain cases, drugs, either alone or used in combina-tion, can even cause brain damage.

Yin and Athletic Performance

Athletes, coaches, and athletic trainers are always looking for an edge, and we are seeing now more than ever a bigger emphasis on the recovery process of sports training. Chronic stress negatively affects an athlete physically, mentally, and emotionally. To perform their best, athletes need each of these areas to be in a positive state. When athletes properly manage stress, they will excel.

Without proper rest, athletes fall into all sorts of traps, including underperformance, burnout, and serious injury. As we explored in the previous section, sympathetic nervous system dominance can lead to serious health consequences that can affect an athlete's performance. For athletes to reach their full potential, they must strive for balance. As I like to say, "Train hard, and rest hard!"

By including yin yoga in your training program, you will strengthen the parasympathetic nervous system. Yin yoga will reduce the production of cortisol and adrenaline, promoting deep relaxation. This relaxation allows the body to sync up the brain–heart–lung connection, which activates diaphragmatic breathing. This increases the flow of oxygen-rich red blood cells, and the body goes into muscle-healing and recovery mode. The body diminishes the lactic acid that has built up through training and reduces inflammation, further reinforcing rest and recovery.

Yin yoga also gives athletes more energy. The stiffer athletes are, the more energy it takes to move their bodies. As their bodies becomes more supple from a yin yoga practice, athletes are able to conserve more energy. This surplus of energy can be used to increase power and stamina.

How about peak brain performance? By switching on the parasympathetic nervous system through yin yoga, you increase blood flow to the cortex and prefrontal cortex regions of the brain. These areas are associated with higher reasoning, better decision making, and mindfulness. Because sports and athletics require a continuous series of decisions that must be made faster than the blink of an eye, optimal brain function is critical for them to be at their best.

Throughout my career, I've been blessed to have various athletes and celebrities reach out in gratitude for my yoga programs. On one occasion, I received a note from A.J. Pollock, an all-star major league baseball player for the Arizona Diamondbacks. He was a first-round draft pick in 2009 out of Notre Dame University. A.J. was coming to town with his team to play the Los Angeles Dodgers and invited me and my wife, Lauren, to a game.

I'll never forget the moment that we stepped onto legendary Dodgers Stadium field with our special on-the-field passes. Fans were pouring into the stands, TV crews were doing their pregame broadcasts, and phenomenal athletes were doing warm-up drills. The energy was electrifying!

A.J. spotted us and trotted over. He expressed tremendous gratitude for my *Ultimate Yogi* program and described it as being one his secret training weapons. In the off-season, he used the stronger power yoga practices, but during the regular season he used the more relaxed practices, especially yin yoga.

But apparently, his secret weapon was no longer a secret. His teammates noticed a difference in his performance and started to inquire. One of his teammates was Paul Goldschmidt. At the time of this writing Paul Goldschmidt, commonly known as Goldy, was one of the best baseball players in the world. He is a multiple MLB All-Star and has won the National League Hank Aaron Award, Gold Glove Award, and Silver Slugger Award.

A.J. called Goldy over to meet us. Immediately, I was struck by how kind and humble he was. Like A.J., he gave thanks for the yoga and also singled out yin yoga for being extra special. He said he had not heard of yin yoga until A.J. turned him onto *The Ultimate Yogi*. After he had been practicing yin for some time, his physical therapists and trainers noticed a huge difference within his body. They noticed a profound shift within his fascia and tissues. Blocked areas of deep tension had released, pain in the body had decreased, and his mobility had improved. For a guy who has been recognized as "America's First Baseman" these results were a big deal.

A.J. then called over the Arizona Diamondbacks third-base coach, Matt Williams. Matt Williams is a former professional third baseman who went to the World Series with the San Francisco Giants and the Cleveland Indians and won the championship with the Arizona Diamondbacks in 2001. A.J. and Goldy had inspired Coach Williams to start doing yoga, which he described as medicine for his aging body. He said that yoga didn't come easy to him, but he always felt tremendously better after doing it, and he was now a solid fan. Then we all had a few laughs about how much yoga can hurt like hell!

Soon after I met Matt Williams, he was hired as the head coach for the Washington Nationals. In 2014, he managed the team to an NL East division title and was named the National League Manager of the Year. One day, I was I scrolling through the news and came across the headline, "Washington Nationals Do Yoga." The article talked about how Coach Williams wanted the entire team to do yoga. As I was reading the article, I couldn't help but smile. Yoga was spreading and was helping teams reach their fullest potential!

Isn't it ironic that when treating a condition, the treatments sometimes have side effects that actually worsen the condition? It seems pretty insane to me. Too many people suffer and lose their lives in an attempt to treat a condition with pharmaceuticals. Although in some circumstances, prescribed drugs are helpful, we also need to be open to a more holistic approach that treats the cause and not just the symptoms.

The number one killer in the United States is heart disease. Personally, I've lost close family members to heart disease, and as I was writing this chapter, my wife's grandfather suffered a near-fatal heart attack. In the past, this condition mostly targeted men, but now heart disease increasingly affects women. According to 2016 data from the Centers for Disease Control and Prevention, one in four deaths each year among women in the United States are caused by heart disease.

High blood pressure is a major precursor for heart disease, which includes heart attack and stroke. Again, according to the Centers for Disease Control and Prevention, one-third of all Americans have high blood pressure and another one-third of Americans suffer from prehypertension, which means they are at high risk for developing high blood pressure (2016a). The number of people afflicted by this disease is staggering.

The science used to discover what causes heart disease has evolved. Back in the 1950s, the main cause of heart disease was said to be high cholesterol levels. Because of this belief, cholesterol-rich and high-fat foods were slandered. Doctors advised their patients to limit or avoid these foods. They also prescribed patients cholesterol-lowering drugs, especially statins. Statins continue to be the most widely prescribed class of medications in the United States.

Galitzer and Trivieri state the following (2015, 355):

> Statin use has done very little to combat heart disease. In fact, a meta-analysis of more than 65,000 patients without a pre-existing condition of heart disease who were prescribed and used statin drugs for a period of five years found that the drugs provided no benefit whatsoever in 98 percent of patients.

According to this study, statins aren't doing their job. Even the placebo effect works significantly better. In addition to their underwhelming effectiveness, statin drugs also have serious side effects. Dr. Galitzer and Trivieri write the following (2015, 355-356):

> The results of these and other studies on statins raise this question: Is cholesterol truly the villain in the story of heart disease? In a word, no. So, if cholesterol isn't the real villain, what is? A growing body of research is attributing it to inflammation, which can be caused by a poor, acidic diet and high levels of stress. When inflammation rises in the body, so does the cholesterol. The cholesterol is part of the human body's defense system to protect it from imbalanced inflammation.

As important as addressing inflammation is, when it comes to heart disease and many other autoimmune disorders, there is another culprit. Dr. Thomas Cowan, who has spent many years researching heart disease and its causes, has found that the primary cause of heart disease and heart attack is the decreased functioning of the parasympathetic nervous system (2014). Dr. Cowan's message is a game changer and a potential life saver.

Dr. Cowan has been joined by a wave of other doctors and scientists who also affirm this belief. The idea that a diminished parasympathetic nervous system plays a significant factor in heart disease was written about in the well-respected medical journals *Circulation* and American *Journal of Cardiology*. An article in *Circulation* stated, "Abundant evidence links sympathetic nervous system activation to outcomes of patients with heart failure (HF). In contrast, parasympathetic activation has complex cardiovascular effects that are only beginning to be recognized" (2008, 863-871). The authors summarized their findings:

> *Autonomic regulation of the heart has an important influence on the progression of HF. Although elevated sympathetic activity is associated with an adverse prognosis, a high level of parasympathetic activation confers cardio protection by several potential mechanisms. These parasympathetic actions on the heart are mediated not only by the direct consequences of cardiac muscarinic receptor stimulation, but also by a multitude of indirect mechanisms.*

Dr. Galitzer and Trivieri explain, "Muscarinic receptors help produce parasympathetic effects, such as a slowed heart rate and increased activity of smooth muscle tissue lining the arteries" (2015, 110). An article published in the *Journal of Cardiology* stated the following (2012, 117-122):

> *In heart failure, it has been recognized that the sympathetic nervous system (SNS) is activated and the imbalance of the activity of the SNS and vagal activity interaction occurs. The abnormal activation of the SNS leads to further worsening of heart failure . . . In conclusion, we must recognize that heart failure is a complex syndrome with an autonomic nervous system dysfunction, and that the autonomic imbalance with the activation of the SNS and the reduction of vagal activity should be treated.*

In the article, "What's the Real Cause of Heart Attacks?," Dr. Cowan explains the chain of events that leads to a heart attack (2014):

> *First comes a decrease in the tonic, healing activity of the parasympathetic nervous system—in the vast majority of cases the pathology for heart attack will not proceed unless this condition is met . . . Then comes an increase in the sympathetic nervous system activity, usually a physical or emotional stressor. This increase in sympathetic activity cannot be balanced because of chronic parasympathetic suppression.*

Dr. Cowan concludes his article by stating, "If heart disease is fundamentally caused by a deficiency in the parasympathetic nervous system, then the solution is obviously to nurture and protect that system, which is the same as saying we should nurture and protect ourselves" (2014).

Before we explore how all this relates to yin yoga, let's also look at another major killer, cancer. Cancer is predicted to overtake heart disease as the number one killer in the United States. Estimates by the American Cancer Society are that almost one in every two men will develop some type of cancer during his lifetime. And for women, it is estimated that one-third will be diagnosed with cancer (2016). Although these estimates are a tough pill to swallow, there is a small shaft of hope. An emerging field, called psychoneuroimmunology, or PNI, is one area of research that shows real promise in the fight against cancer. PNI puts an emphasis on the mental, psychospiritual, and emotional factors that make people susceptible to cancer. It also explores which factors can contribute to better patient outcomes.

PNI says that the effect of stress on the autonomic nervous system, along with the onslaught of chronic inflammation, have a massive impact on the survival of cancer cells. Dr. Holloway, who has had a lot of success using his NuCalm technology to work with cancer patients says the following (quoted in Galitzer and Trivieri 2016, 86):

> *Cancer isn't something you catch. Cancer develops when your body's immune system is not taking care of rogue cells. Everybody develops cancer cells every day, but your oncogene (a mutation of a gene involved in normal cell growth) sends in a little protein message that tells the cancer cells to die. This is called programmed cell death, or apoptosis. It's when this system, which is part of the immune system, is not working that you can end up with cancer.*

We have explored in depth the consequences of chronic stress, sympathetic dominance, and chronic inflammation. We know that the cause of diseases that kill millions of people per year across the globe are linked to deficient parasympathetic activity. So, where does yin yoga fit into the picture? Well, it is relevant in so many ways. This is one of the most important messages I want to convey in this book. The intention behind yin is slowing to allow the body's natural intelligence to achieve balance. In your yin yoga practice, you diminish the sympathetic nervous system and engage the parasympathetic nervous system. The stress hormones of cortisol and adrenaline decrease, and the feel-good hormones of serotonin and dopamine increase. Inflammation lowers. The limbic brain, associated with fight or flight, is downregulated by the positive activation of the prefrontal cortex. Now the entire brain is fully integrated. The body's rest-and-repair mechanism is fully activated. The connective tissues of the body are hydrated, strong, and durable. This is the key to health and longevity.

So much suffering, sickness, and death could be prevented by living a life of greater balance. Yin yoga along with a healthy diet, exercise, proper lifestyle, meditation, and quality sleep will tremendously increase your quality of life. Yin yoga is not a luxury; it is a necessity.

> *"The doctor of the future will give no medicine but will interest his patients in the care of the human frame, in diet and the cause and prevention of disease."* —Thomas Edison

This chapter presented a lot of information on what happens deep in the body. My hope is now that you understand the science behind yin yoga and its benefits, you are even more inspired to practice. Practicing yin yoga keeps the connective tissues and nervous system healthy so that your brain can communicate effectively with all the cells. This proper flow of communication ensures that you maintain an optimal state of vitality. The next phase of our journey together explores the poses of yin yoga.

Dr. Jeremy Brook

Dr. Jeremy Brook is a Los Angeles chiropractor, yogi, and movement special-ist. In 2001, Dr. Brook founded The Life Center Chiropractic, a unique healing oasis that incorporates the disciplines of chiropractic medicine, spinal correc-tive protocols, yoga, and other movement art forms to make sure the spine, body, and mind are aligned.

T.E. The first question is when we do yin yoga, which tissues are we exposing?

J.B. It's a simple answer because everything is completely interconnected. There's really no separation if you really want to get down to it. There's no start and there's no finish. So, I say everything. But if you want to get a little bit more technical, you're going to be stretching the connective tissue. If you want to break it down even further, you're talking about stretching fascia, you're going to be stretching muscles, you'll be involving tendons, and you'll be involving the ligaments. Depending on how intense your stretch is, especially in yin, you're going to be expanding or compressing the organs as well.

T.E. When you are holding a yin pose, how long does it take to get into the connective tissue?

J.B. One of my teachers from chiropractic school, named Dr. Robert Cooper-stein, had a published paper on this topic and he said five minutes. If you want to get into the fascia, and the connective tissue, then you have to relax. If your muscles are tense, then you're not really able to hit the fascia. Five minutes is the maximum amount of time you need to hang out in a shape to create that type of fascial change. That being said, he also did say that it was beneficial to hang out in that posture for about 90 seconds to two minutes. But it appears that the two-minute to five-minute period is where you're probably going to get the greatest benefit. And these days I'd say it's probably closer to the five-minute mark just because everyone's living more in a sympathetic state. I think for the psychological benefits, in addition to the tissue benefits, five minutes is the magic number.

T.E. What's your favorite yin yoga pose?

J.B. My favorite yin yoga pose has evolved. [laughter] I want to say it's shoelace pose. I love that one because not many poses in yoga really focus on putting the hips into internal rotation, it tends to be an externally rotated dominant practice.

T.E. What's your least favorite yin yoga pose?

J.B. I'm going to say caterpillar. [laughter]

T. E. Why should people make the time for yin yoga?

J.B. A lot of people are attracted to the yang energy. They want the pump. I think that once people realize that, then they know they need to add more of a parasympathetic-style aspect to their life. A lot of the diseases that plague mankind, especially in the West, are the diseases of overexcitement, where you have way too much tension and inflammation and toxicity accumulating inside of the body. We need to tap into the part of the system that restores, that regenerates, that deals with our growth and development, that allows for our immune system to get turned on, and that allows for our energy system to get turned on. Yin is how you reboot, restart your system, get your energy levels back up, and shift out of fight or flight. And there's a part of me that wants to just say, "Don't be such a fool; there's another part of your body that needs to be fed and nourished, and you're only doing the hard pounding, the charging, and your body needs a chance to refresh."

Or we could just say it's good for your joints and it's good for your ligaments. It's going to open you up, you're going to be more flexible, and you'll have better performance in various aspects of your life. Because the people who are just pounding with the yang only, are tapping into half of the story, and they're missing out on the other half.

CHAPTER 5
POSES OF YIN YOGA

"Take care of your body. It's the only place you have to live."

—Jim Rohn

Up to this point we have explored the background and context of yin yoga. Our journey has taken us through the history, philosophy, subtle anatomy, and the science of yin yoga. In this chapter, we get into the actual yin poses. Many of the poses have been passed down through the lineage of yin yoga, and others are new additions that expand the practice. Different teachers may call the same pose by different names. In fact, you might recognize that some poses from hatha yoga have a different name in the yin yoga tradition. For each pose, I have listed the name, suggested duration, benefits, risks and contraindications, alignment points, modifications, and other options. My intention is to give you as much information as possible to set you up for success within your practice (more detail on your personal practice will be presented in chapter 7). Before we explore the yin poses in depth, let's take a look at the Three Laws of a Yin Pose.

Three Laws of a Yin Pose

The way that we exercise muscle is different from the way that we exercise connective tissue. If you want to strengthen a muscle such as a biceps, then you stress it by doing repetitive, strong, and explosive movements. For example, pick an appropriate weight and do 8 to 12 biceps curls. This exercise will break down the muscle tissue. After rest, the body will repair and rebuild the muscle, assuming you give it proper nutrition. Then the next time you do the exercise after the muscle has recovered, the movement will be more efficient and the weight easier to curl. The natural Tao of the body knows how to adapt. This example describes a yang style of exercise to address the yang nature of the muscles.

The connective tissues however, are characterized by yin and need to be exercised in a yin manner. So, what makes a yin yoga pose? Instead of a fast, dynamic movement, the connective tissues respond to a slow, sustained hold. Practitioners of yin yoga typically hold a relaxed posture for three to five minutes, which exerts a positive stress on the connective tissues as a way to trigger the body's natural repair response. This leads to a stronger, more durable, and supple body. This method then triggers a set of events that makes the connective tissues stronger, longer, and more durable. Because the connective tissue is found in nearly every structure of the body, this is a boon for your overall health and performance capabilities.

No matter what yin pose you do, the following three laws will always be present. Anytime you work with these three guidelines, you know that you are working within the realm of yin. Remember these now and forever.

Find Your Edge

When you enter into a posture, you first look for your edge. This is a wall of resistance that keeps you from proceeding farther. Trying to force and push

YIN POSES

Now that we've discussed the "The Three Laws of a Yin Pose," let's unpack the details of the yin poses. Keep in mind that the pictures you see of my wife, Lauren, and me are just examples of how the poses *can* be done. The photographs are meant to serve as general guidelines; however, all bodies are different. You might be more flexible or restricted. Each of us has our own unique anatomy and history. Do your best to follow the alignment points and modify as you need to. If your pose looks different than the picture, that is OK. Always trust the wisdom of your body. All right, here we go!

through this wall isn't yin; it is yang. Imagine yourself gently leaning into that wall. Depending on the situation, the wall could indicate tissue tightness or it could indicate anatomical limitations. If anatomy, rather than tissue tightness, is the limitation then your range of motion has been fully expressed. During the posture, aim for positive discomfort and not bad pain.

Find Stillness

Once you find your edge and settle into the sweet spot in the pose, strive for stillness. Stillness is synonymous with yin. Finding stillness doesn't mean that you can't fine-tune and adjust your position. It just means that if you need to move, do it mindfully. Frequently, our movements are unconscious and reactive. If we are in a pose and experience discomfort, many of us try to distract ourselves from what we are feeling. This could arise as an itch, a desire to adjust clothing, or the temptation to pick at our fingernails. You wouldn't believe the number of people I've seen in a yin pose become enamored with their nails. If you need to, make a mental note to set up a mani-pedi appointment, and then come back to yin practice. Eliminate unnecessary, fidgety behavior.

Let Time Flow

Yin yoga is not about quantity; it's about quality. You may not execute nearly as many poses as in a flow class, but that's not the point. The point is to spend a substantial amount of time in each pose in a deep, concentrated way. The strength of yin yoga comes from this flow of time. The longer you hold, the deeper you go. The deeper you go, the deeper you heal. The deeper you heal, the better you will feel. So being patient is to your benefit. Developing patience is an added bonus of your yin yoga practice. The more patience you have, the less stressed and anxious you will be. So how long do you hold? The magic window of time for holding a yin pose is usually three to five minutes.

CATERPILLAR POSE

Suggested Duration

3-5 minutes

Benefits

This cooling posture targets the back of the body, providing both attention to the muscles along the spine and a healing touch to the abdominal organs.

Risks and Contraindications

This pose is contraindicated for people with back pain caused by herniated or bulging discs.

Alignment Points

- Begin in a seated position and extend both legs straight.
- Reach the arms overhead, draw the shoulders down, and fold forward from the crease of the hips, grasping the outer edges of the feet or legs.
- Draw the heart forward and elongate the spine. Draw the belly up and in as the front ribs draw down and elongate the torso.
- Bow the forehead down, allowing the head and neck to relax.

Modifications and Other Options

If you have lower-back pain or tightness in the hamstrings, modify the pose by bending the knees, placing a folded blanket under the sitz bones, or performing the pose using a strap around the soles of the feet.

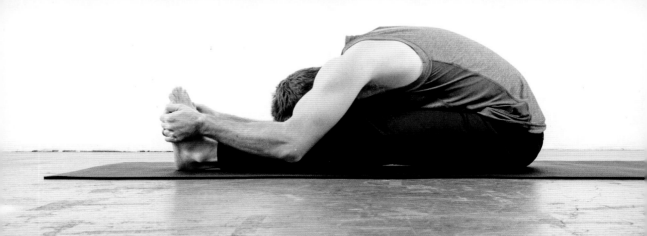

BUTTERFLY POSE

Suggested Duration

3-5 minutes

Benefits

This pose stretches the hips, inner thighs, and groin muscles and can help alleviate sciatica.

Risks and Contraindications

Modify or work into the pose with caution if you have low-back pain or knee injuries.

Alignment Points

- Begin in a seated position, drawing the soles of the feet together and then drawing the heels toward the body. Open the knees away from each other.
- Grab the outer edges of the feet as you roll the outer hips to the floor.
- Fold over, allowing your spine and back to release.
- You can keep the hands on the outer edges of the feet or reach the arms out in front along the floor.

Modifications and Other Options

- If you have low-back pain, place a blanket or prop under the sitz bones to elevate the hips.
- If you have knee issues, place a block or prop under the outer hips.
- If you have a neck injury or excessive tension, you can support the head with a block or bolster under the forehead.

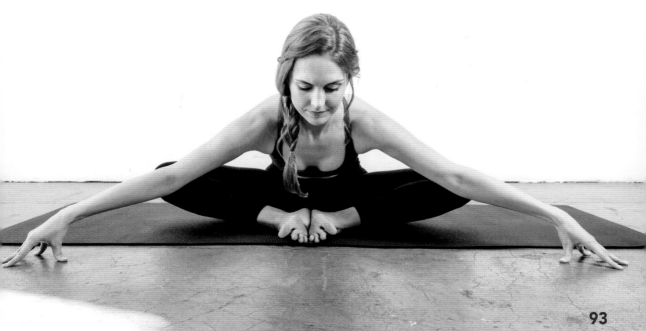

HALF-BUTTERFLY POSE

Suggested Duration

3-5 minutes

Benefits

This calming and cooling posture elongates the spinal muscles, hamstrings, and glutes.

Risks and Contraindications

Modify this pose or proceed with caution if you have a history of knee pain.

Alignment Points

- Begin in a seated position and extend one leg straight forward, with the extended foot gently flexed.
- Bend the opposite knee, and press the sole of the foot into the inner upper thigh of the extended leg.
- Reach the arms overhead, draw up through both sides of the waist, and fold from the crease of the hips while lengthening the sternum forward.
- Grasp the foot or shin of the extended leg, and relax in the forward bend.
- Repeat on the other side.

Modifications and Other Options

- If you have knee issues, place a blanket under the bent knee for support.
- For more of an inner-leg stretch, rotate the torso so it is facing between the thighs and then crawl the hands out along the floor (1).
- For a great side stretch, turn the chest to face the same direction as the bent knee, rolling the top ribs open to the sky. One arm reaches along the inseam of the extended leg while the other arm reaches upward or outward (2).

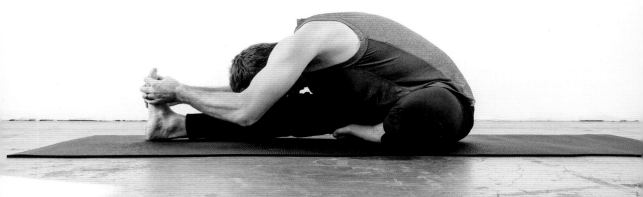

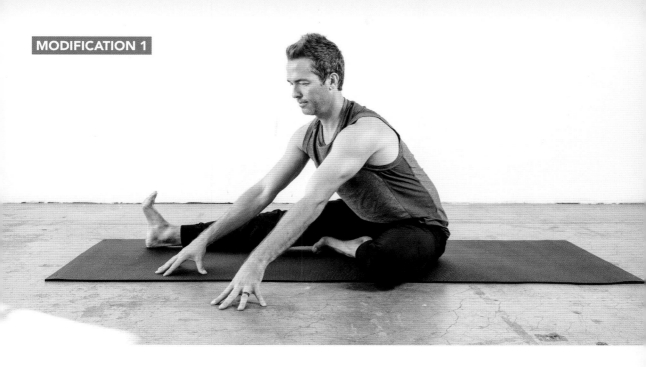

MODIFICATION 1

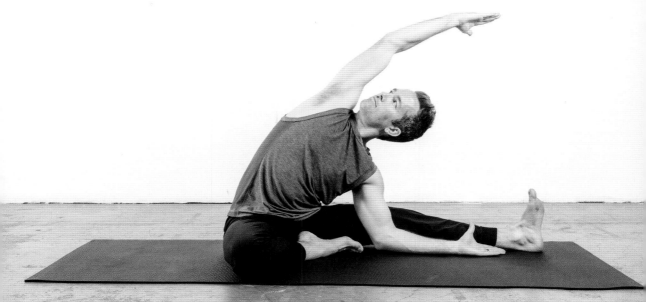

MODIFICATION 2

DRAGONFLY POSE

Suggested Duration

3-5 minutes

Benefits

This calming and cooling posture lengthens the back of the body, provides traction for the spine, opens the hamstrings, and stretches the inner thighs.

Risks and Contraindications

This pose is contraindicated for those with groin injuries, back pain, or bulging or herniated discs.

Alignment Points

- Begin in a seated position and spread the legs apart.
- Gently flex the feet.
- Rotate the outer thighs to keep the knees pointing straight up.
- Align the torso directly over the sacrum and root the sitz bones into the ground.
- Extend the torso forward while bringing the arms in front along the floor, or reach the hands out and grab the legs or feet.
- Draw the shoulder blades down and away from the ears.

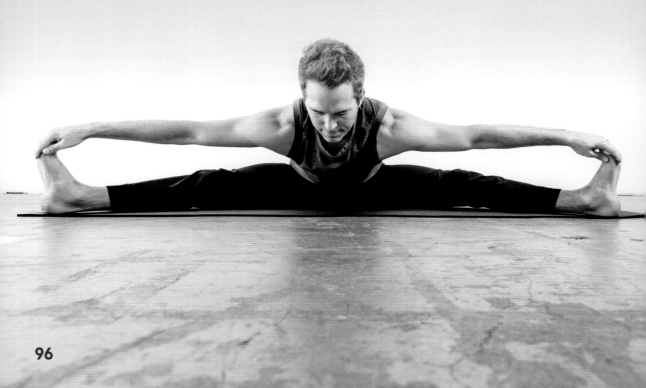

Modifications and Other Options

- If you have a history of back pain, place a folded blanket under the sitz bones and proceed cautiously or remain upright.
- Feel free to target one leg at a time by bringing the torso toward one side and reach the hands out while grabbing the foot or shin (1). Allow the chest to melt toward the leg. Repeat on the other side.

MODIFICATION 1

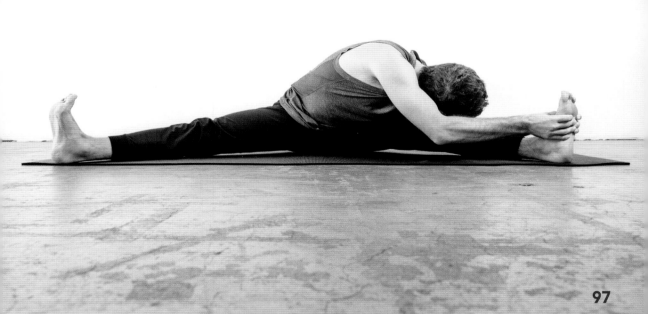

FROG POSE

Suggested Duration

2-5 minutes

Benefits

This pose stretches the hips and groin.

Risks and Contraindications

This pose is contraindicated for those with hernias. It can be modified if you have knee pain.

Alignment Points

- Begin on all fours and spread the knees wider than the hips.
- Flex the feet and spread the feet wider than the knees.
- Lower the forearms to the mat and place the elbows under the shoulders. Either place the hands on the mat and spread the palms, or interlace the fingers.
- Press the hips back and tilt the tailbone forward.
- Keep the shoulders soft and draw the crown of the head forward. Gaze toward the floor, keeping the cervical spine aligned with the rest of the spine.

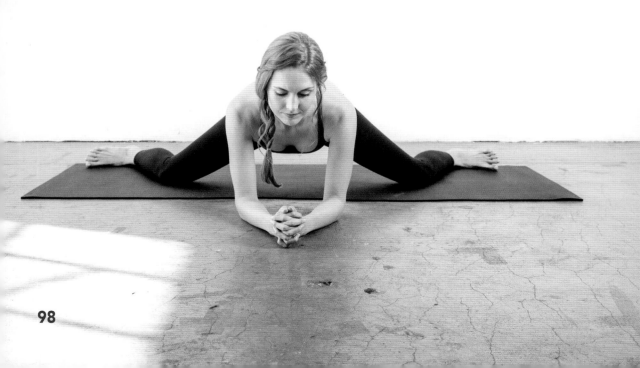

Modifications and Other Options

- If you feel pressure in the knees, place a blanket under them to provide padding.
- If the pose is too intense, bring the toes in and lift the hips higher (1).
- Placing a bolster under the chest can add a softer quality.

MODIFICATION 1

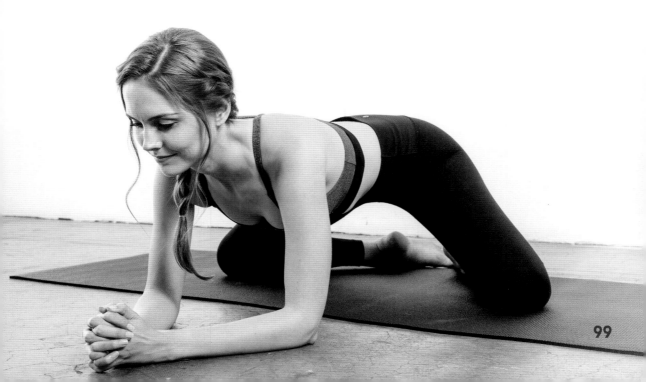

99

HALF-FROG POSE

Suggested Duration

2-4 minutes

Benefits

This pose provides a deep stretch for the groin and inner thighs, provides stimulation for the knee of the bent leg, and stretches the top of the foot of the bent leg.

Risks and Contraindications

Modify this pose if you have sensitive knees or low-back issues.

Alignment Points

- Begin in a seated position.
- Extend your right leg out straight, bend your left back by your outer left hip, and open your left knee toward the left side of your yoga mat. Ideally, you want a 90-degree angle at the inner thighs.
- Slide your whole body to the right side of your yoga mat so that the outer right leg lines up with the edge of the mat. Make sure that your inner left knee is supported by the cushion of the mat.
- Turn your chest to face between the inner thighs.
- Crawl your hands forward and out until you find a stretch.
- Repeat on the other side.

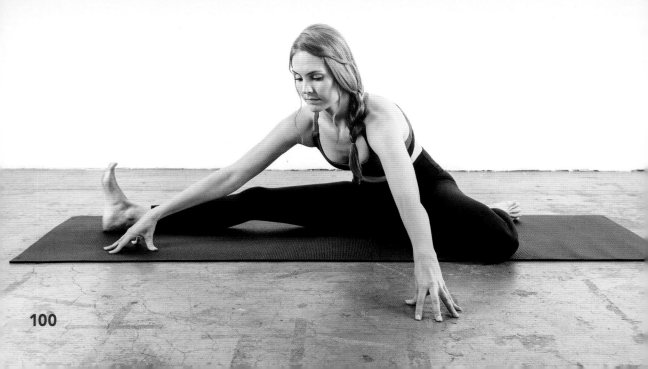

Modifications and Other Options

- If you have sensitive knees, modify or replace with half-butterfly (page 94).
- If you have low-back issues, keep the spine as straight as possible.
- If this pose is too intense, place a prop under the hip of the extended leg to take the pressure off the opposite knee. You can also place a blanket or extra padding under the same knee.
- For more of a hamstring and spine stretch, crawl your torso toward the extended leg. Reach the hands out and allow the chest to drape over the thigh (1).
- Bring the left arm inside the extended leg, and reach the right arm to the sky. Open the top of the chest, and reach the right arm toward the left foot. Flexible students can grab the outer edge of the left foot and roll the top ribs open to the sky (2). This variation provides more of a stretch for the muscles along the side of the torso.

MODIFICATION 1

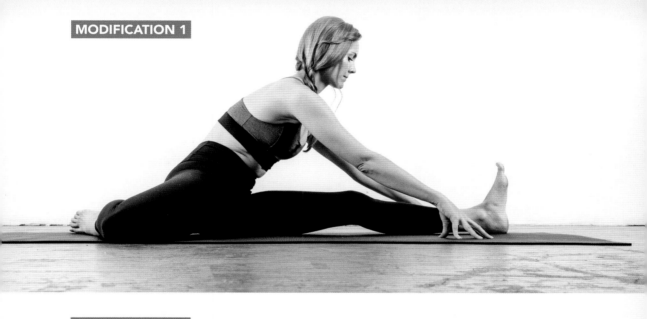

MODIFICATION 2

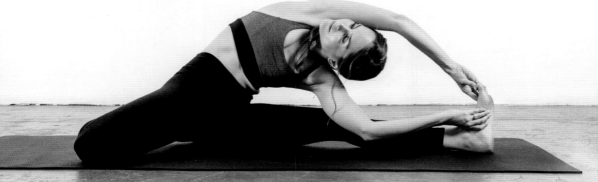

CHILD'S POSE

Suggested Duration

3-5 minutes

Benefits

This is a cooling and calming pose that activates the nervous system's relaxation response. This pose stretches the hips and lower back and the tops of the feet.

Risks and Contraindications

Modify the pose if you have a knee injury or tight hips.

Alignment Points

- From a kneeling position, bring the big toes together and separate the knees wider than the torso.
- Fold forward from the crease of the hips and place the forehead on the floor.
- Place the arms by the sides or bring them forward while bending the elbows and relaxing the shoulders.
- Drop the hips back toward the heels.
- Close the eyes and relax the head and neck.

Modifications and Other Options

- If you have knee issues or tight hips, place a rolled blanket in the fold of the legs behind the knees for additional support.
- Place a block or bolster under the forehead if the head doesn't comfortably rest on the floor.
- If you have tightness in the shoulders, either bring the arms behind you or bend the elbows.

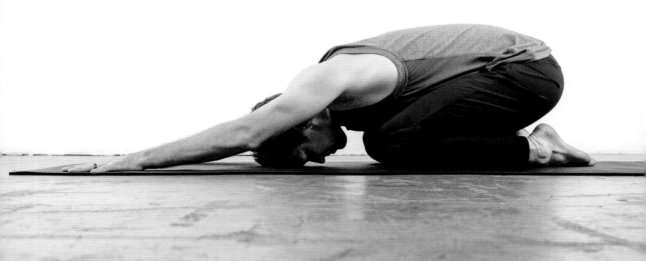

MELTING HEART

Suggested Duration

2-5 minutes

Benefits

This pose is a backbend that also stretches the shoulders.

Risks and Contraindications

This pose is contraindicated for people who have neck or shoulder issues. Also, if you feel tingling or numbness in the hands, come out of the pose.

Alignment Points

- Begin on all fours.
- Crawl the arms out in front of you, spreading the hands a little wider than the shoulders.
- Wrap the outer arms down and spiral the inner arms up in external rotation to broaden across the upper back and shoulders.
- Keep the hips above the knees.
- Allow the chest to relax down toward the floor.
- Rest the forehead on the floor.

Modifications and Other Options

- Place a blanket under the shins and feet for comfort.
- Rest the forehead on a block to support the neck.

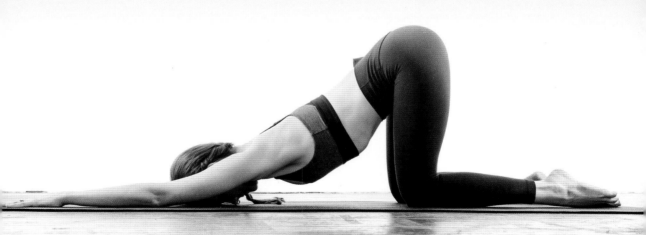

CAMEL POSE

Suggested Duration

2-3 minutes

Benefits

This pose opens the chest and shoulders and stretches the thighs, hip flexors, and front of the body. It can be used as a backbend for students who are pregnant.

Risks and Contraindications

This pose is contraindicated for students with lower-back pain, neck injuries, high blood pressure, heart disease, or a history of stroke. Modify the pose if you have knee pain.

Alignment Points

- Begin by kneeling, stack the shoulders over the hips, and place the hands on the hips.
- Press the shins and tops of the feet into the mat. Roll the pinkie toes down and point the toes straight back.
- With the knees hip-distance apart and the sitz bones over the knees, roll the inner thighs back.
- Place the hands on the low back and lengthen the tailbone toward the floor.
- Lift the back ribs as the heart rises toward the ceiling and roll the shoulders back, pressing the shoulder blades toward the back ribs.

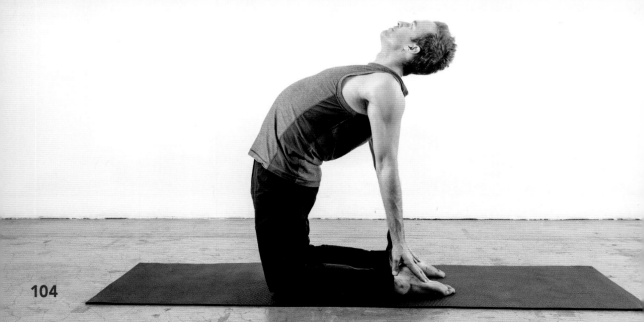

- Lift the gaze toward the ceiling, keeping the cervical spine in alignment with the rest of the spine.
- If you have enough flexibility in the back and enough stability in the pose, you may release the hands to the heels.

Modifications and Other Options

- If you have knee pain, sensitivity, or injury, use a folded blanket under the knees for support.
- If you are close to placing the hands on the heels but still straining, tuck the toes under to elevate the heels. If there is still strain, then return the hands to the lower back.
- For a one-armed camel, place your right hand on top of the right heel and reach the left arm toward the sky (1). Repeat on the other side. Tuck the toes under to modify.

MODIFICATION 1

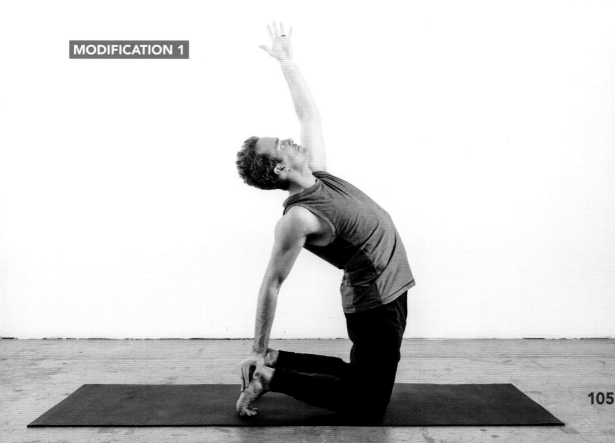

105

THREAD-THE-NEEDLE SHOULDER STRETCH

Suggested Duration

2-3 minutes

Benefits

This pose opens the shoulder and chest and provides a relaxing spinal twist.

Risks and Contraindications

Be gentle if you have a history of neck pain. Also, if you experience tingling or loss of sensation in the hands, come out of the stretch.

Alignment Points

- Begin on all fours and extend one arm toward the sky, stretching through the top chest.
- Lower the arm and thread it under the opposite arm, releasing the outer shoulder onto the floor.
- Repeat on the other side.

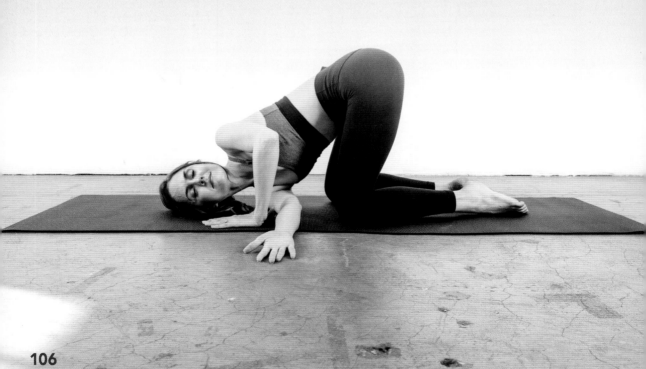

Modifications and Other Options

- Place a blanket under the knees, shins, and feet for comfort.
- The hand positioned in front of the face can slide forward toward the top of the mat for more of a shoulder stretch in that arm (1).
- The hand positioned in front of the face can also reach around behind the back and either grab the inner thigh or rest on the sacrum (2).

MODIFICATION 1

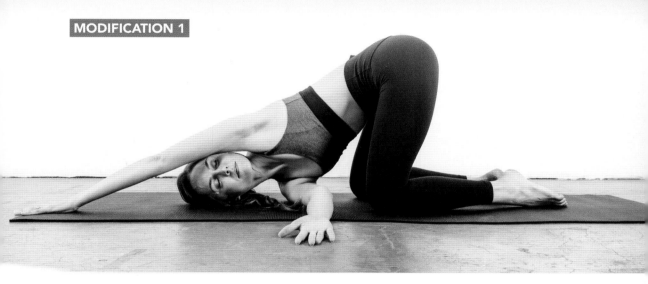

MODIFICATION 2

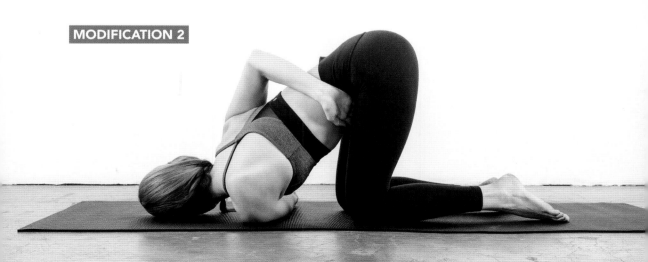

DANGLING STANDING FORWARD BEND

Suggested Duration

2-3 minutes

Benefits

This is a great standing yin pose that yields to gravity, providing decompression for the spine, shoulders, and elbows. It also provides a gentle release for the hamstrings and the back of the knees.

Risks and Contraindications

Avoid this pose if you have high blood pressure, glaucoma, or vertigo. Modify it if you have low blood pressure or lower-back pain. If you feel tingling or loss of sensation in the hands, release the arms and simply hang like a rag doll.

Alignment Points

- Begin in a standing position, with the feet hip-width apart.
- Reach the arms over the head and then fold the torso out over the legs.
- Grab opposite elbows with opposite hands to create a box or frame around the head.
- Allow the head and neck to completely relax.
- Gently sway side to side or lightly bounce up and down.

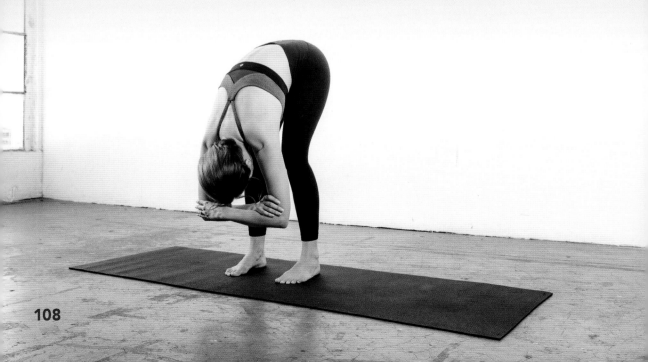

Modifications and Other Options

- For more of a shoulder stretch, bring the hands around to the lower back and, while interlacing the fingers, draw the arms toward straight (1).
- If you have low blood pressure, exit mindfully by rolling up slowly and continuing to breathe.
- If you have lower-back pain, bend the knees as much as you need to soften the intensity of the stretch.

MODIFICATION 1

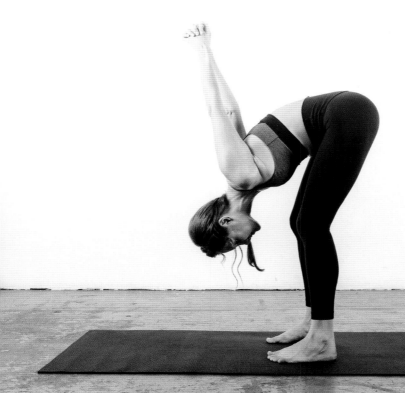

109

SQUAT

Suggested Duration

2-3 minutes

Benefits

This pose stretches the hips; lengthens the lower back; and strengthens the pelvic floor, legs, and calves. It also improves focus and can relieve back pain.

Risks and Contraindications

This pose is contraindicated for students with knee or hip pain.

Alignment Points

- Begin in a dangling standing forward bend (page 108), and then step to the side so the feet are wider than the hips and the toes are turned out.
- Allow the tailbone to melt toward the floor until the sitz bones are a few inches above the mat.
- Press the outside edges of the feet to the floor while lifting the inner arches.
- Bring the hands together in prayer and press the elbows into the knees and the knees into the elbows.

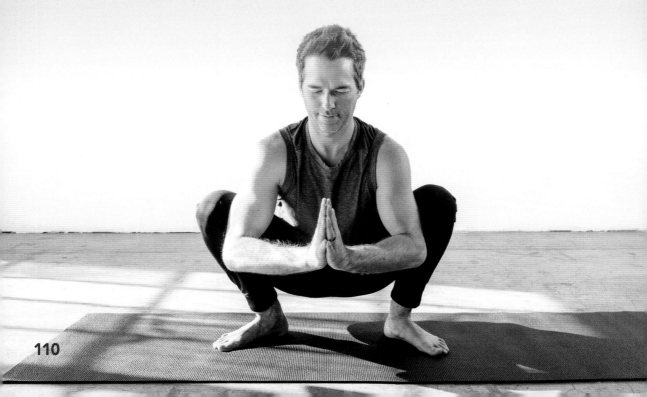

- Lift the sternum away from the hips and lengthen the back of the body.
- Gently relax the shoulders away from the ears and spread the shoulder blades.
- Gaze ahead or allow the chin to slightly tilt down, lengthening the back of the neck.

Modifications and Other Options

- Place a block under the sitz bones for support.
- If the heels lift off the floor, spread the feet wider. If the heels still do not touch floor, place a rolled blanket or yoga mat under the heels for support.
- For a bonus shoulder and chest stretch, reach the left arm around the front of the left shin and reach the right arm around behind the back (1). If you're able, grasp your fingers together and open the right side of your chest (if shoulders are tight, you can always use a strap). Repeat on the other side.

MODIFICATION 1

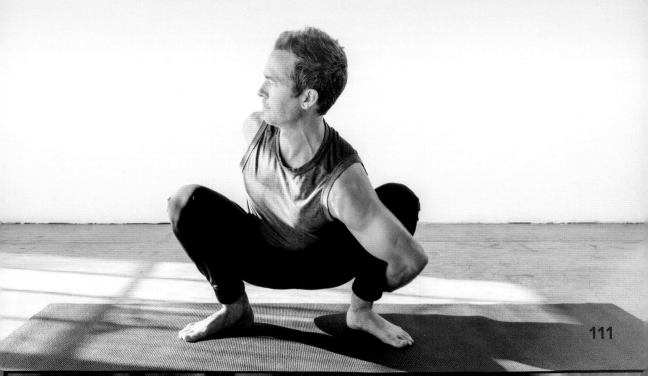

111

TOE SQUAT POSE

Suggested Duration

2-3 minutes

Benefits

This pose targets the tissues in the feet and toes.

Risks and Contraindications

Modify this pose if you have sensitive feet or lower-back pain.

Alignment Points

- From a standing position, bend the knees into a squat while allowing the toes to lift off the floor as you sit back on the heels.
- Put your hands on the floor for balance and let the knees gently release onto the floor.
- Bring your hands to prayer, keeping the toes tucked under and feeling the stretch in the feet.
- Exit the pose with mindfulness by reversing your movements.

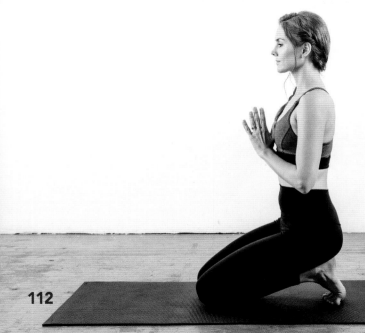

Modifications and Other Options

- If you have pain in the knees, place a blanket under them for comfort.
- If you feel too much sensation in the feet, keep your hands on the floor or on blocks to alleviate some of the pressure.
- If you have lower-back pain, keep the spine vertical or in a slight tilt forward.
- For an even deeper stretch, bring your hands behind you on the floor, turn the fingers away from you, and then lean back into a backbend (1).

MODIFICATION 1

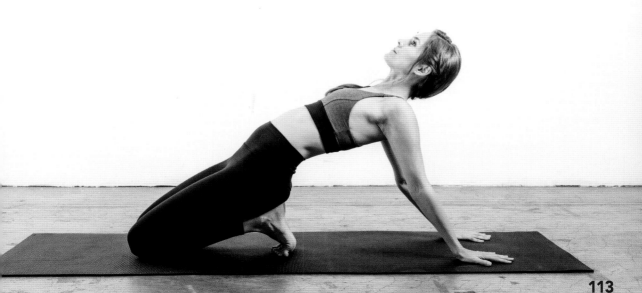

113

ANKLE STRETCH

Suggested Duration

2-3 minutes

Benefits

This pose targets the ankles and tops of the feet.

Risks and Contraindications

If you have tight ankles (like runners!), ease into the stretch with caution. If you feel sharp pain in the knees, then ease out of the pose.

Alignment Points

- Begin in a kneeling position, sitting on the heels.
- Place both hands on top of the knees.
- Gently lean back until the shins and knees lift off the floor.
- Maintain the length of the spine so that you resist collapsing through the spine.
- Don't let the head fall back and overextend the neck.

Modifications and Other Options

- Place a blanket under the feet for added comfort.
- Doing the pose without lifting the knees off the floor still provides a solid stretch (1).
- If balance is an issue, place the hands on the floor next to the body or on top of blocks for support.

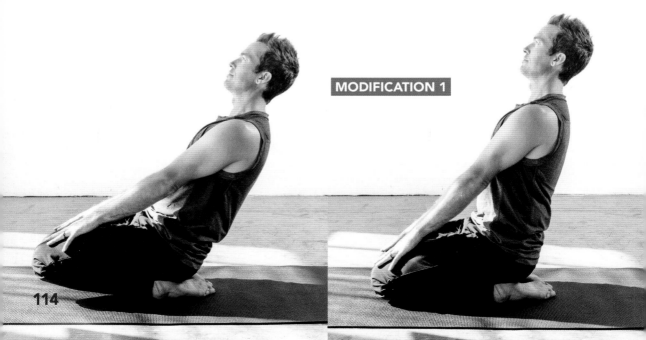

MODIFICATION 1

SADDLE POSE

Suggested Duration

3-5 minutes

Benefits

This pose provides a stretch for the tops of the feet, ankles, and thighs and a positive compression for the sacrum, which promotes a healthy lower back. It also maintains the health of the knees.

Risks and Contraindications

This pose is contraindicated if you have an acute knee injury. If you have stiff ankles or lower-back pain, do not recline.

Alignment Points

- Begin on all fours and crawl your hands back by your knees.
- Bring your big toes together and spread your knees outward.
- Sit back on your heels.
- If you feel comfortable doing so, recline onto your forearms or relax all the way onto your back. If reclining, the knees should remain in contact with the ground.

Modifications and Other Options

- Place a blanket under the tops of the feet and shins for comfort.
- If you recline back, place a bolster under your back and head for support.

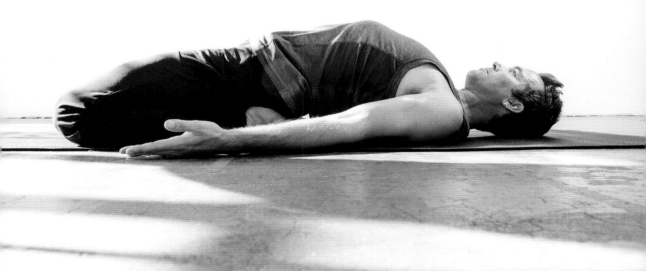

HERO POSE

Suggested Duration

3-5 minutes

Benefits

This pose provides a stretch for the tops of the feet, ankles, and thighs and a positive compression for the sacrum, which promotes a healthy lower back. It also maintains the health of the knees as long as you ease into it with caution.

Risks and Contraindications

Modify the pose if you have a stiff or sensitive back, or choose saddle pose instead (page 115). If you have stiff ankles or lower-back pain, do not recline.

Alignment Points

- Begin on all fours and crawl the hands back to the knees.
- Bring the knees together and spread the feet wider than the knees.
- Sit back between the ankles and rest the hands comfortably on top of the thighs.
- If you feel comfortable enough to do so, recline onto the forearms or all the way onto the floor. If reclining, the knees should remain in contact with the ground.
- The arms can rest by the sides, or the hands can rest on the ribs, or the elbows can be bent at 90 degrees and the palms facing the sky as in the cactus position.

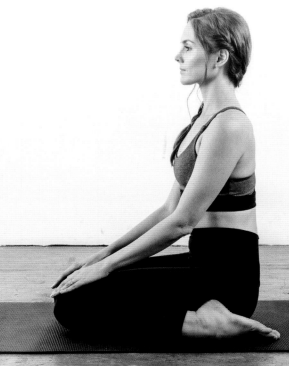

Modifications and Other Options

- If you have stiff or sensitive knees, place a block under the sitz bones.
- Place a blanket under the tops of the feet and shins for comfort.
- If you recline, place a bolster under your back and head for support.
- For a half-hero pose, keep one foot bent back by the outer hip while the other leg extends straight out (1). Repeat on the other side.
- For a deeper variation, bend one knee toward the sky, keeping the sole of the foot flat on the floor (2) or pull the thigh in toward the chest (3).

MODIFICATION 1

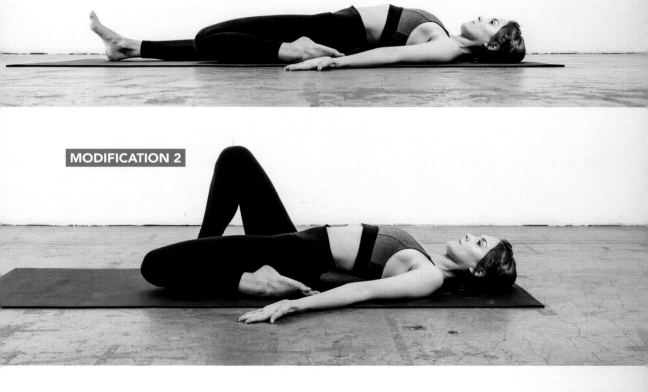

MODIFICATION 2

MODIFICATION 3

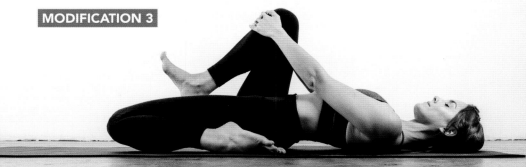

EASY SEATED POSE

Suggested Duration

2-5 minutes

Benefits

This is a calming pose that teaches proper posture and promotes internal reflection. It is a common posture used for pranayama and meditation practices. Easy seated pose is a modification for the fire log pose (page 126).

Risks and Contraindications

Modify the pose if you have knee pain, tight hips, or low-back pain.

Alignment Points

- Start in a seated position and root the sitz bones to the mat.
- Cross the shins and allow the ankles to rest under the knees with the outer edges of the feet in contact with the floor. Actively flex the feet to protect the knees.
- Stack the shoulders over the hips and align the crown of the head over the shoulders, keeping the chin parallel to the floor.
- Gaze ahead, relax the shoulders back, and draw the front of the ribs down, with the belly pulling in slightly.
- Place the hands of top of the thighs or rest them comfortably in the lap.

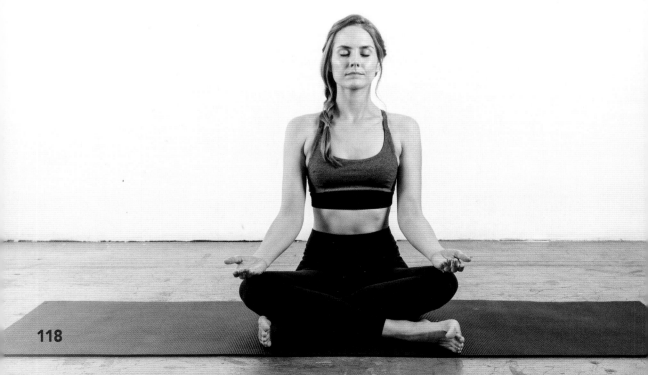

Modifications and Other Options

- If you have lower-back pain, tight hips, or sciatica, sit on a block or a folded blanket in order to raise the hips higher than the knees for support.
- Fold the torso over and down for a stretch into the hips (1). This is a modification for fire log pose (page 126).
- While maintaining easy seated pose, you can stretch the upper-body tissues using the lateral neck stretch (page 154), forward neck stretch (page 153), cow face arms (page 156), reverse prayer (page 157), and eagle arms (page 160).

MODIFICATION 1

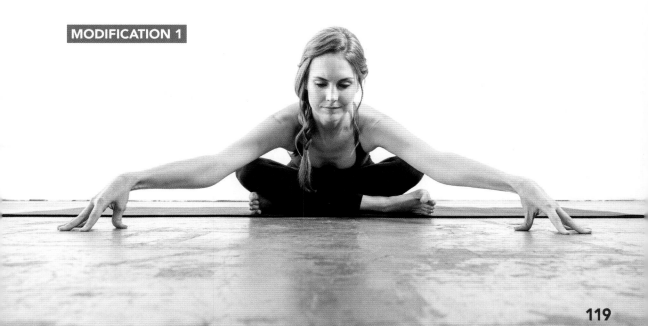

EASY SEATED TWIST

Suggested Duration

2-3 minutes

Benefits

This simple twist is appropriate for students of all levels and benefits the spine and gently massages the organs in the abdomen.

Risks and Contraindications

Modify this pose if you have lower-back pain, tight hips, or sciatica.

Alignment Points

- Begin in easy seated pose (page 118) and cross the right shin in front of the left shin.
- Place the left hand directly behind the sacrum, and keep the spine straight and tall.
- Place the right hand on the left knee and roll the shoulders back and down.
- Draw the right hip back so that both hips point directly forward. This will ensure that the twist is created through the movement of the shoulder girdle.
- As the sternum lifts, draw the front of the ribs down and the belly back toward the spine.
- Depending on the health of the neck, shift the gaze over the front or back shoulder and keep the chin parallel to the floor.
- Repeat on the other side.

Modifications and Other Options

If you have lower-back pain, tight hips, or sciatica, sit on a block or a folded blanket in order to raise the hips higher than the knees for support.

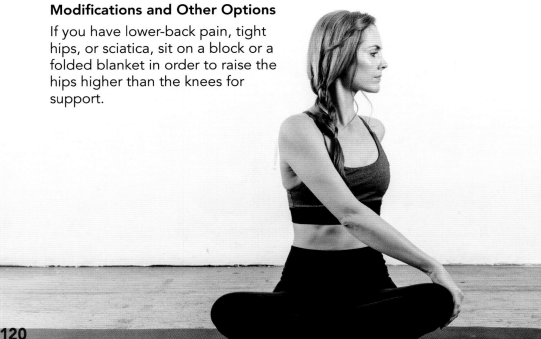

SEATED DIAMOND POSE

Suggested Duration

3-5 minutes

Benefits

This is a calming and cooling posture that stretches the outer hips and the spine, especially the lower back. It is also a great posture if you are pregnant.

Risks and Contraindications

Modify this pose if you have sciatica, knee issues, or lower-back problems.

Alignment Points

- Begin in a seated position.
- Bring the soles of the feet together, with the toes forward and the knees opened outward.
- Slide the feet forward, further than in butterfly pose (page 93), until the lower body is shaped like a diamond.
- Bring the hands to the feet or ankles.
- Extend out through the spine and fold forward into the stretch, allowing the elbows to flare out.

Modifications and Other Options

- If you experience discomfort in the lower back, place a blanket or cushion under the sitz bones to elevate the hips.
- If you feel pain in the knees, place blocks or cushions under the outer hips for support.
- Placing a block under the forehead helps to relax the neck muscles.

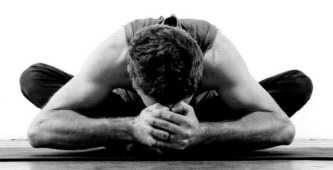

DEER POSE

Suggested Duration

3-5 minutes

Benefits

This pose stretches the hips. For some students, this pose is a great alternative to sleeping swan (page 123).

Risks and Contraindications

If you have knee pain, don't bend forward too far.

Alignment Points

- Begin in a seated diamond (page 121).
- Move your left leg behind you, keeping the knee bent and the foot positioned behind the hip.
- Allow the front shin to move toward the top edge of your yoga mat.
- Let your weight naturally lean to the left.
- With your hands on the floor in front of you, allow your torso to fold over toward the floor.
- Repeat on the other side.

Modifications and Other Options

- If you experience pain in the front knee, put a cushion under that hip for support.
- For a more calming effect, place a bolster under the torso or a block under the forehead.

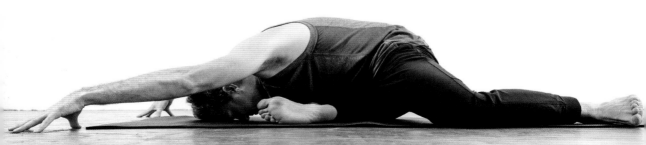

SLEEPING SWAN

Suggested Duration

3-5 minutes

Benefits

This pose stretches the hips and groin.

Risks and Contraindications

This pose is contraindicated for students with lower-back pain and those with hip, knee, or ankle pain or injuries. Modify the pose if you have tight hips or an ankle injury or experience pain.

Alignment Points

- Begin on all fours and bring one shin forward, resting it toward the top of the mat. Flex the front foot to activate the shin and protect the knee.
- Extend the back leg straight, keeping the top of the foot flat on the floor and the toes spread.
- Align the shoulders directly over the sacrum, relax the shoulders back, and spread through the front of the chest as both sides of the waist lift. Keep the pelvis facing forward.
- Slowly lower the chest toward the floor and keep the sternum moving forward to lengthen the spine. Use the forearms for support or rest the chest on the floor.
- Soften the gaze or gently close the eyes.
- Repeat on the other side.

Modifications and Other Options

- If you have tight hips and are unable to sustain the pose without strain, place a block, folded blanket, or bolster under the front hip for support. You can also place a block under the back upper thigh.
- If you have knee or ankle injuries or pain, perform reclining pigeon (page 140) or deer pose (page 122) as a modification.

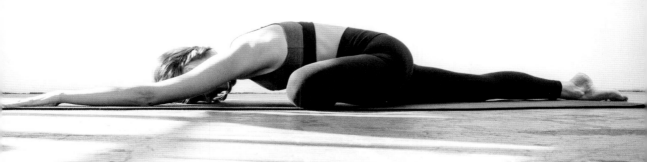

SHOELACE POSE

Suggested Duration

3-5 minutes

Benefits

This pose provides a stretch through a unique internal hip rotation.

Risks and Contraindications

Modify the pose if you have hip, knee, or lower-back pain.

Alignment Points

- Begin on all fours, and cross one knee in front of the other. Lean forward and hug the inner thighs toward each other while spreading the feet wider than the hips.
- Sit the hips between the heels and press the tops of the feet into the floor. Rotate the pinkie toes toward the mat and point the feet toward the back of the mat.
- Anchor the sitz bones and lift both sides of the waist while softening the front of the ribs downward.
- Draw the crown of the head toward the ceiling, keeping the chin parallel to the floor, and relax the shoulders back.
- Rest the hands on the inner arches of the feet and allow the torso to tilt forward until you find your edge.
- Repeat with the other leg on top.

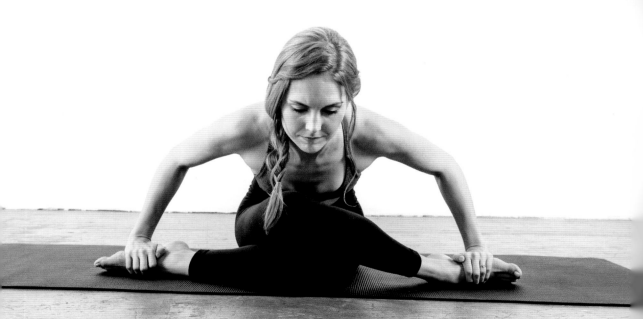

Modifications and Other Options

- If you have pain in the knees or hips, place a block under the sitz bones for support.
- For an added side stretch, reach your hand on the floor to the left when the right leg is on top. Bring the right arm up and over, expanding across the right ribs (1). Repeat on the other side.
- For half shoelace, extend your left leg toward straight with the right leg bent over the top. Reach your hands forward, grabbing your left leg or foot, and coming into a forward bend (2). Repeat on the other side.

MODIFICATION 1

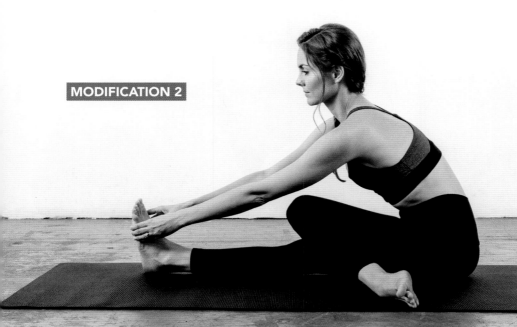

MODIFICATION 2

FIRE LOG POSE

Suggested Duration

3-5 minutes

Benefits

This pose stretches the outer hips and groin.

Risks and Contraindications

This pose is contraindicated for students with knee pain or sciatica.

Alignment Points

- Begin in a seated position, bend one knee and align the shin parallel to the front of the mat, and flex the foot.
- Bend the opposite knee and align the shin directly on top of the bottom shin, allowing the top foot to rest directly on top of the bottom knee. Flex the top foot.
- Align the shoulders directly over the sitz bones.
- Place the hands by the hips and lift the sternum, gazing directly ahead.
- Sweep the arms overhead and reach the hands forward, folding from the crease of the hips.
- Throughout the pose, lengthen the back of the neck and keep the cervical spine aligned with the rest of the spine.
- Keep the sitz bones firmly rooted to the floor and relax the shoulders back.
- Repeat on the other side.

Modifications and Other Options

- If your knees and shins do not stack comfortably, perform easy seated pose (page 118).
- Place a block under the forehead to support the weight of the skull.

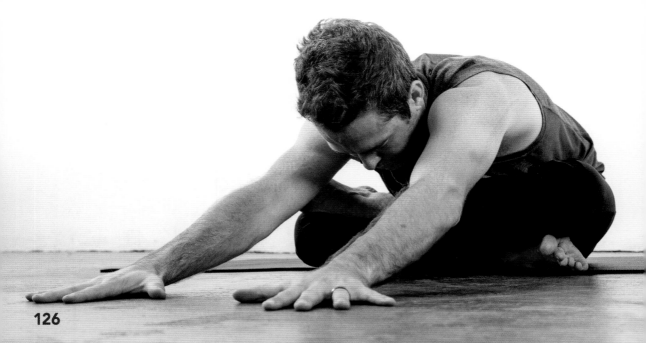

SPHINX POSE

Suggested Duration

3-5 minutes

Benefits

This pose is a gentle backbend that supports overall spine health and provides awareness of the shoulder girdle.

Risks and Contraindications

This pose is contraindicated for students who are pregnant.

Alignment Points

- Begin on the belly and slide the forearms forward, aligning the elbows directly under the shoulders, middle fingers pointing ahead, and all four corners of the hand pressing evenly into the mat.
- Draw the heart forward by pressing down and then into the forearms and drawing the elbows back.
- Press the pubic bone into the floor and lengthen the lower back by tilting the pelvis toward the face.
- Draw the shoulders away from the ears, relax the tops of the feet onto the floor, and roll the inner thighs up and outer thighs down.
- Feel the lower belly lift, bringing the backbend into the upper back.
- Gaze directly ahead or allow the chin to tilt slightly down.

Modifications and Other Options

- To relax the neck, place a block under the forehead for support.
- If you experience discomfort as the frontal hip points press into the floor, place a blanket under that area to add extra cushion.

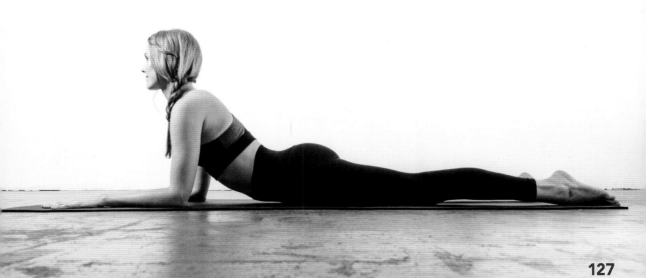

DRAGON POSE

Suggested Duration

2-5 minutes

Benefits

This pose stretches the psoas, hip flexors, and quadriceps and it can be good for relieving sciatica. It is also beneficial for the pelvis.

Risks and Contraindications

Modify this pose if you have knee pain or tight ankles.

Alignment Points

- Begin on all fours with the spine in neutral position and step one foot forward, stacking the front knee directly above the front ankle.
- Allow the back knee to rest on the mat.
- Slide the knee along the mat so it is behind the sitz bones.
- Draw the chest forward and broaden the collarbones while relaxing the hands on top of the front thigh.
- Repeat on the other side.

Modifications and Other Options

- If the back knee feels like it's grinding into the floor, place a blanket under it to provide extra cushion and comfort.
- To lessen the intensity of the pose, place the hands on top of blocks for support.
- To increase the intensity, use low dragon pose by bringing both hands to the inside of the front foot and sliding the front foot a little toward the outside edge of the mat. Bend both elbows, allowing the torso to drop down toward the floor (1). If needed, place a block under the forearms for support.

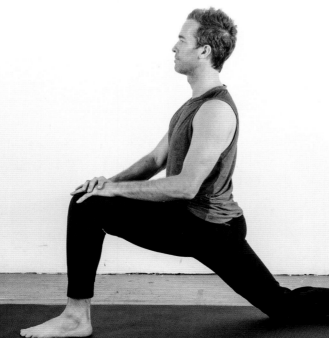

- For an even deeper stretch, move into low angled dragon pose by rolling onto the outer edge of the front foot, letting the knee flare outward. Keeping the torso low, crawl away from the foot and toward the opposite edge of the mat. Reach the arms out and allow the chest and head to relax down toward the floor (2). Repeat on the other side.

MODIFICATION 1

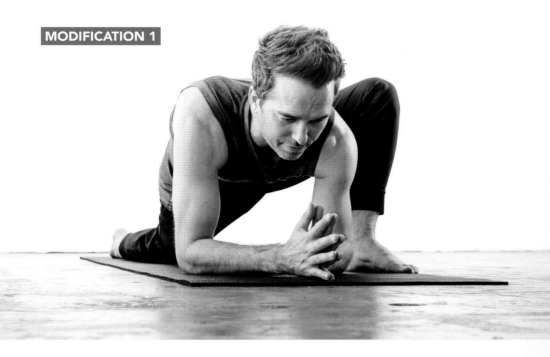

MODIFICATION 2

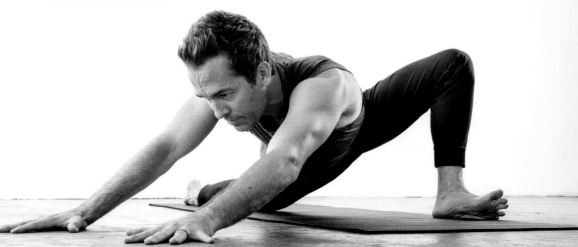

HALF SPLITS

Suggested Duration
2-5 minutes

Benefits
This pose stretches the hip flexors, groin, hamstrings, and quadriceps.

Risks and Contraindications
This pose is contraindicated for students with hernias or knee, hip, or lower-back pain.

Alignment Points
- Begin in dragon pose (page 128) and extend the front leg forward while pulling the hips back.
- Balance on the front heel, with the toes facing upward.
- Rest the hands on the floor or blocks or reach a hand out and grab the front foot.

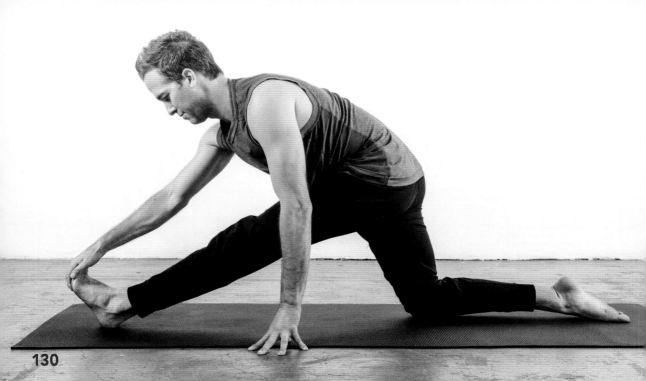

Modifications and Other Options

- If you experience discomfort in the back knee, place a blanket under it to provide extra cushion.
- Place blocks under both hands to lessen the intensity.
- For more intensity, use full splits by sliding the back leg toward the back of the mat, keeping the shin and top of the foot pressing into the mat for stability. Then, slide the front heel forward and square the hips toward the front of the mat, allowing the torso to fold forward and the hands to rest on the floor (1). Repeat on the other side. If necessary, place a block under the front hamstrings for support.

MODIFICATION 1

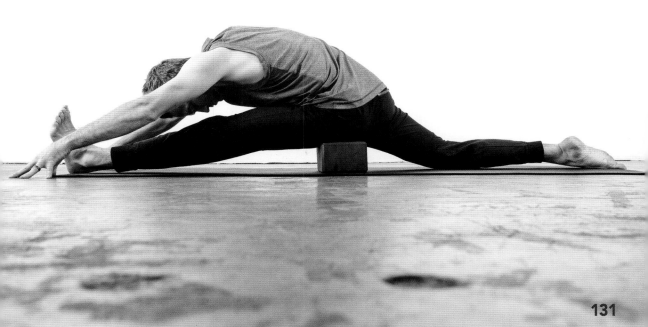

131

RESTING BELLY POSE

Suggested Duration

3-5 minutes or longer

Benefits

This pose triggers the parasympathetic nervous system, helping to alleviate stress and promote relaxation and calmness.

Risks and Contraindications

This pose is contraindicated for students who are pregnant. Modify if you have neck issues.

Alignment Points

- Lie on your belly.
- Bring your hands on top of each other as if you were creating a pillow, allowing the elbows to open out.
- Allow the forehead to rest on top of the hands.
- Close the eyes or soften the gaze.
- Relax and let gravity pull you into the floor.

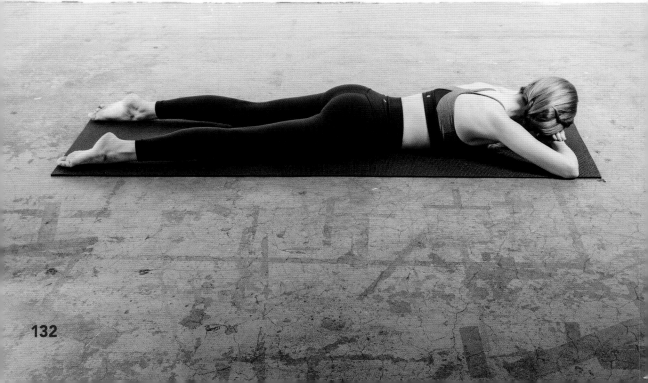

Modifications and Other Options

- If you are looking for a side neck stretch, turn the head to the side. Repeat on the other side.
- If you feel discomfort in the lower abdomen, place a blanket under this area.
- Gently rocking side to side can provide a stretch through the lower back.
- As an alternative, students who are pregnant should try lying on their left side with their knees slightly bent and their hands under the side of the face (1).

MODIFICATION 1

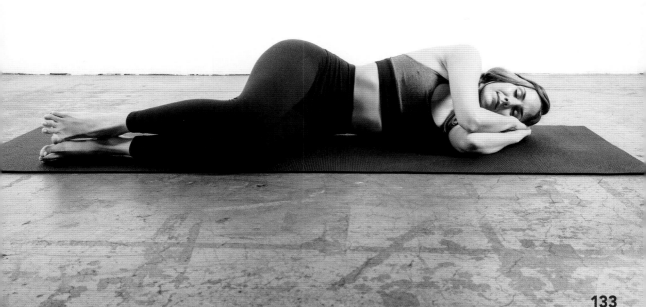

SEAL POSE

Suggested Duration

3-5 minutes

Benefits

This pose is a healing backbend that counters the constant force of gravity on the spine. It provides a good stretch to the abdominal muscles, and helps to open the respiratory channels for improved breathing.

Risks and Contraindications

Students who have back issues should avoid or modify this pose. Pregnant students should not press the belly into the floor.

Alignment Points

- Begin on your belly and come into sphinx pose (page 127) by sliding your forearms forward until the elbows are under the shoulders.
- After taking a few breaths, slide your hands out and away from the body, opening them up a little wider than the shoulders.
- Rotate your fingers slightly outward and press into your hands as you elevate your chest toward the sky and wrap the outer shoulders back.
- Slide your shoulders down and back to avoid creating tension in the neck.

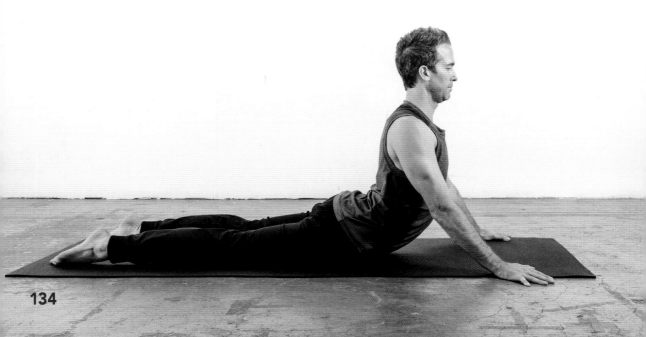

Modifications and Other Options

- If you feel pressure on the frontal hip points and pubic bone, place a blanket under that area for comfort.
- For less intensity, remain in sphinx (page 127), which provides the same effects but in a gentler way.
- To deepen the stretch, bend the knees, bringing the feet in toward the body (1).

MODIFICATION 1

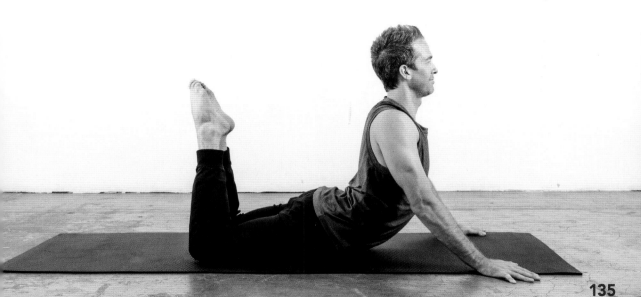

135

RECLINING BUTTERFLY

Suggested Duration

2-4 minutes

Benefits

This pose activates the relaxation response, which can help lower blood pressure, reduce stress, relieve sciatica, and alleviate discomfort during menstruation, menopause, and pregnancy. It stretches the hips through external rotation.

Risks and Contraindications

Modify the pose if you have tight hips, knee pain, or sciatica.

Alignment Points

- Begin by reclining on your back.
- Bring the soles of the feet together, allowing the knees to gently release outward.
- Allow the arms to extend out away from the body and rotate the palms toward the sky.
- Relax the shoulders down and back.
- Relax and feel free to close the eyes.

Modifications and Other Options

- If you have tight hips, knee pain, or sciatica, position blocks or bolsters under the hips and knees for support.
- Other options for arm position include bringing the arms into cactus, where the elbows are bent 90 degrees and the palms face the sky, or resting one hand on the belly and the other hand on the chest.

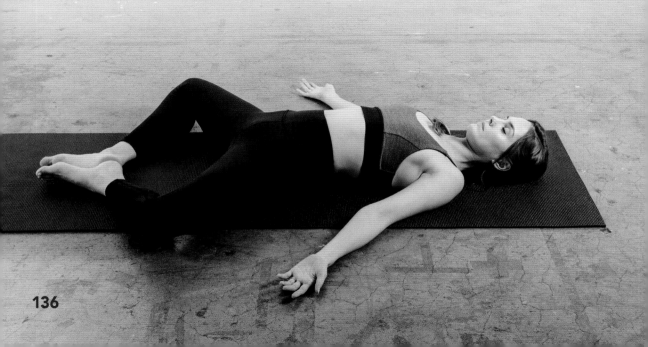

RECLINING TEEPEE

Suggested Duration

2-4 minutes

Benefits

This pose activates the relaxation response, which can help lower blood pressure, reduce stress, relieve sciatica, and alleviate discomfort during menstruation, menopause, and pregnancy. For students who experience discomfort in the hips, this pose is a great alternative to reclining butterfly (page 136).

Alignment Points

- Begin by reclining on your back.
- With the feet flat on the floor, spread the feet the width of your yoga mat and allow the knees to fall in toward each other for support.
- Allow the arms to extend out and away from the body, and rotate the palms toward the sky.
- Relax the shoulders down and back.
- Relax and feel free to close the eyes.

Modifications and Other Options

Other options for arm positions include bringing the arms into cactus, where the elbows are bent 90 degrees and the palms face the sky, or resting one hand on the belly and the other hand on the chest.

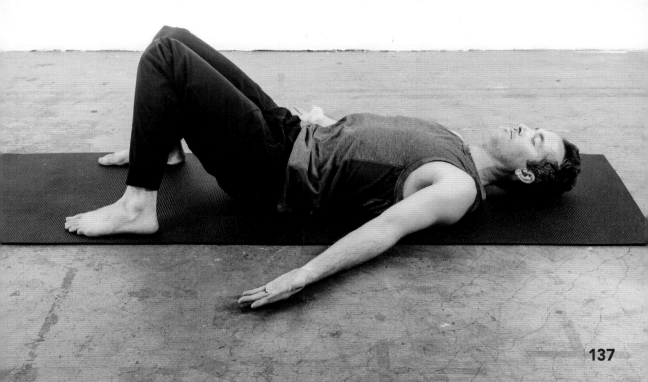

RECLINING TREE

Suggested Duration

2-4 minutes

Benefits

This pose provides an external hip stretch and opens the chest and lungs. It also promotes calmness and relaxation.

Risks and Contraindications

Modify or exit the pose if you experience discomfort in the hip.

Alignment Points

- Begin by lying on your back and extending one leg straight.
- Bring the opposite foot up to the inner thigh of the extended leg and allow the bent knee to release off to the side.
- Open the arms to the side or bring them into cactus, where the elbows are bent 90 degrees and the palms face the sky.
- Repeat on the other side.

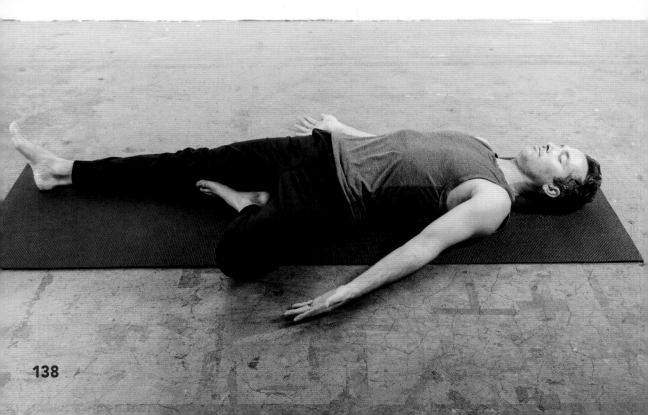

Modifications and Other Options

- If you experience discomfort in the hip or the knee, place a cushion under that hip for support.
- For a deeper stretch, place one foot on the upper thigh of the extended leg for a half-lotus variation (1).
- To promote greater relaxation, drape a blanket across the belly.

MODIFICATION 1

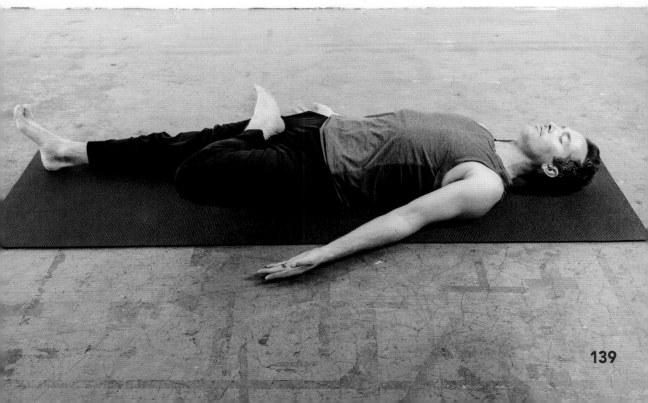

RECLINING PIGEON

Suggested Duration

2-4 minutes

Benefits

This pose is a cooling hip opener appropriate for students at all levels, especially those with a history of knee injuries.

Risks and Contraindications

This pose is contraindicated for students who are pregnant. Modify the pose if you have knee injuries or tight hips.

Alignment Points

- Begin by reclining on your back with the knees bent and the feet flat on the floor, hip-width apart.
- Cross the right ankle on top of the opposite thigh and actively flex the right foot.
- Draw the left thigh toward the chest and reach the hands around the shin.
- Wrap the right thigh forward while drawing the left thigh in.

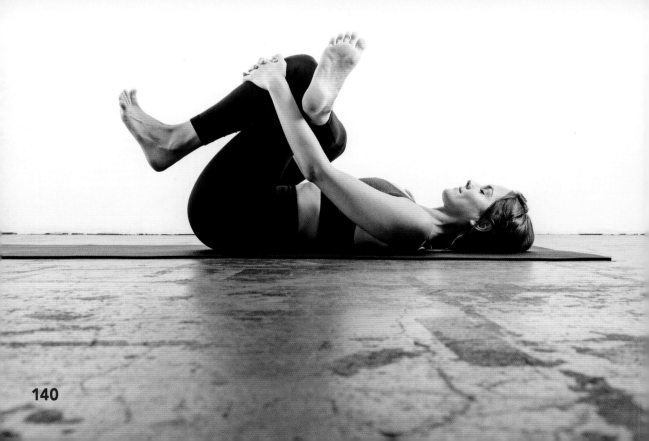

- Rest the back of the head on the mat and stretch the crown of the head toward the back of the mat.
- Relax the shoulders down and back and broaden through the upper chest.
- Soften the gaze.
- Repeat on the other side.

Modifications and Other Options

- If you have knee issues, hold the back of the thigh instead of the front of the shin.
- If you have tight hips, use a strap around the front of the shin or back of the thigh to help draw the knee in.
- Another option for students with tight hips is to keep the left foot flat on the floor while placing the right ankle on top of the right thigh and gently flexing the right foot (1). Repeat on the other side.

MODIFICATION 1

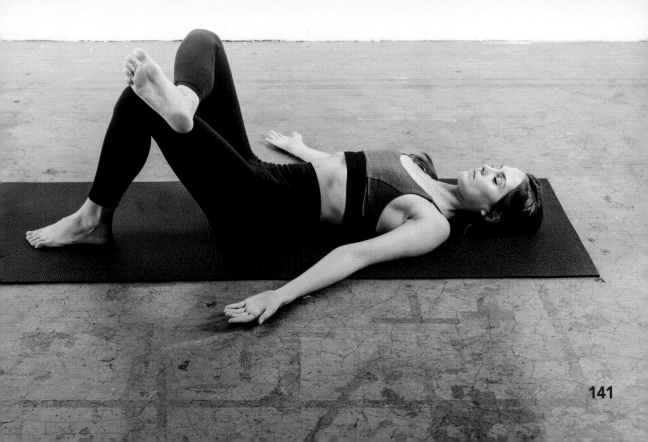

STIRRUP POSE

Suggested Duration

3-5 minutes

Benefits

This pose stretches the hips and groin.

Risks and Contraindications

This pose is contraindicated for pregnant students. Modify the pose if you have a neck injury or pain.

Alignment Points

- Begin by reclining on your back and hug the knees into the chest. Slide the hands down the legs and grab the outside edges of the feet. Lift the soles of the feet up to the sky.
- Open the knees wider than the torso, but continue hugging them toward the ribs.
- Lower the knees toward the floor while flexing the feet toward the sky and stacking the ankles directly above the knees.
- Spread the collarbones wide and let the back of the head rest comfortably on the floor.
- Move the chin slightly away from the chest, gently curving the cervical spine away from the mat.
- Direct the gaze toward the sky.

Modifications and Other Options

- If you have tight hips, hold the backs of the thighs or the ankles instead of the feet.
- If you have a neck injury, place a folded blanket under the head for support.
- For half-stirrup pose, extend one leg out straight and bend that knee, keeping the foot flat on the floor. A personal favorite is to bring the bottom leg on the floor into the same position used in reclining butterfly (page 136).

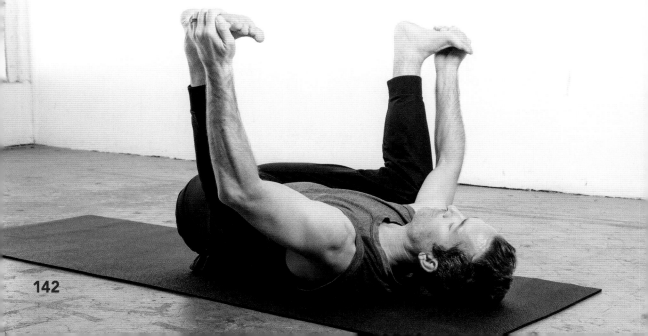

SUPPORTED BRIDGE

Suggested Duration

3-5 minutes or longer

Benefits

This backbend pose is cooling and passive. For students with a history of herniated discs, it can help rebuild the lumbar spine.

Risks and Contraindications

Modify this pose if you have lower-back or neck pain or neck injury.

Alignment Points

- Begin by lying on the back, with the soles of the feet flat on the mat. Lift the hips, and place a block at the lowest height under the sacrum, with the long edge perpendicular to the spine rather than along the length of the spine.
- Rest the arms by the sides with the palm facing up.
- Keep the feet hip-distance apart and allow the inner thighs to spiral down as the knees continue to point directly ahead.
- Soften the shoulders and the front of the ribs, and relax the front of the body.

Modifications and Other Options

- If you have a history of back pain, use a bolster or a low block that does not aggravate the pain. If you feel comfortable deepening the stretch, adjust the block so it is taller.
- Variations include bringing the arms into cactus position, with the elbows bent at 90 degrees and palms facing up, or resting one hand on the belly and the other hand on the chest.

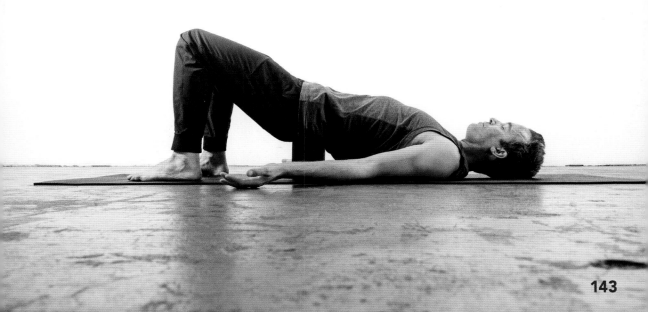

BANANA POSE

Suggested Duration

2-5 minutes

Benefits

This pose stretches the muscles along the side of the torso through lateral spinal flexion.

Risks and Contraindications

Students with lower-back issues should be careful not to flex too far. Modify the pose if you experience discomfort in the shoulders.

Alignment Points

- Begin by lying on your back.
- Slide both the head and the feet toward the left side as you slide the hips to the right, creating a crescent shape through the body.
- Place the right leg over the top the left leg and then gently grab the right wrist with the left hand.
- Repeat on the other side.

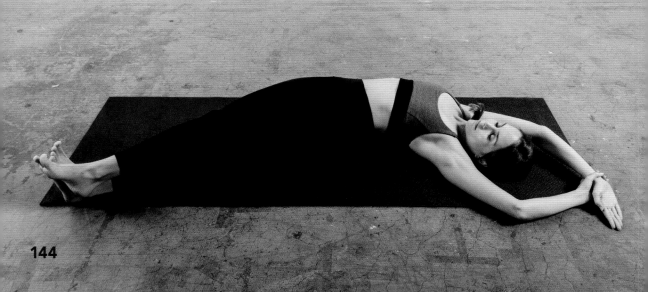

Modifications and Other Options

- If you feel discomfort in the shoulders, either grab opposite elbows with opposite hands to frame the head (1) or bring the arms to cactus variation, where the arms are bent at 90 degrees and the palms face up.
- If you feel numbness in the hands, rest them on the front ribs or exit the pose sooner.

MODIFICATION 1

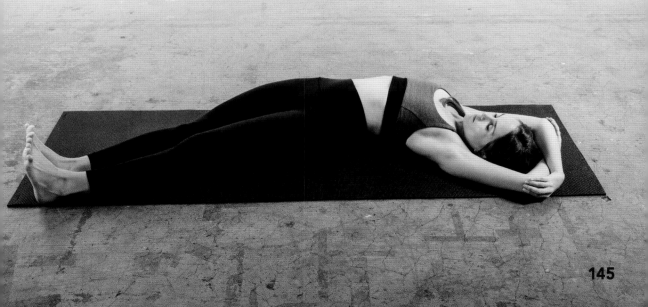

145

SNAIL POSE

Suggested Duration

2-5 minutes

Benefits

This pose is a calming posture and it massages the abdominal muscles. It is also a shoulder opener that relieves tension through the upper back.

Risks and Contraindications

This pose is contraindicated for students with high blood pressure, history of stroke, a hernia, acid reflux, neck pain, or a history of neck injuries.

Alignment Points

- Begin by lying on your back, with the arms by the sides and palms facing down.
- Extend the legs up and over the head toward the back of the mat. If the toes do not touch the floor, bring the hands to the lower back for support. If the toes do touch the floor, the palms may stay flat on the mat or the hands may interlace to help draw the shoulders under. You may place the tops of the feet flat on the floor, reaching the toes back to stretch the shins.

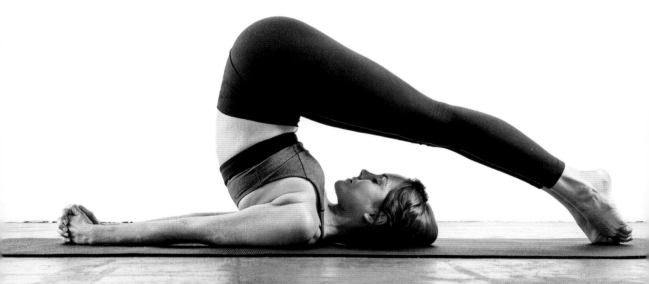

- Stack the hips directly over the shoulders and draw the shoulder blades toward each other, keeping the neck long and maintaining the natural curve of the cervical spine.
- Direct the gaze upward as the back of the head presses into the floor.

Modifications and Other Options

- Place a blanket under the shoulders to support the neck.
- Bend the knees and reach back with the hands, grabbing onto the outer edges of the feet for a deeper stretch (1).

MODIFICATION 1

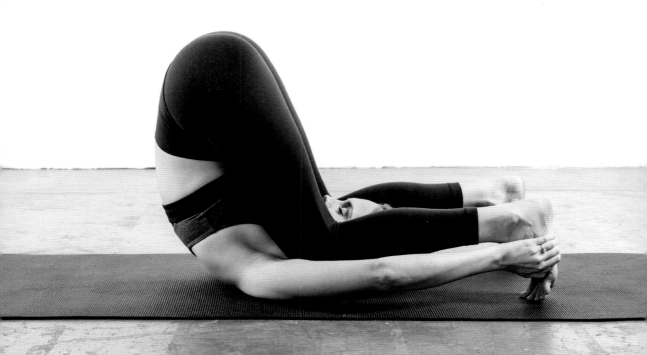

RECLINING TWIST

Suggested Duration

2-4 minutes

Benefits

This simple but sweet pose provides a release across the lower back and a gentle massage to the belly organs.

Risks and Contraindications

Modify the pose if you have neck issues or discomfort in the shoulders.

Alignment Points

- Begin on your back and draw both knees into the belly.
- Keeping the right knee in, extend the left leg straight along the floor. Reach the right arm to the right.
- Place the left hand on the outer right knee, and guide the knee all the way over into the twist.
- Repeat on the other side.

Modifications and Other Options

- If you have neck issues, look straight up or perhaps in the same direction as the bent knee.
- If you have discomfort in the shoulder, bend the elbow into cactus arm (elbow bent at 90 degrees and palms facing up).

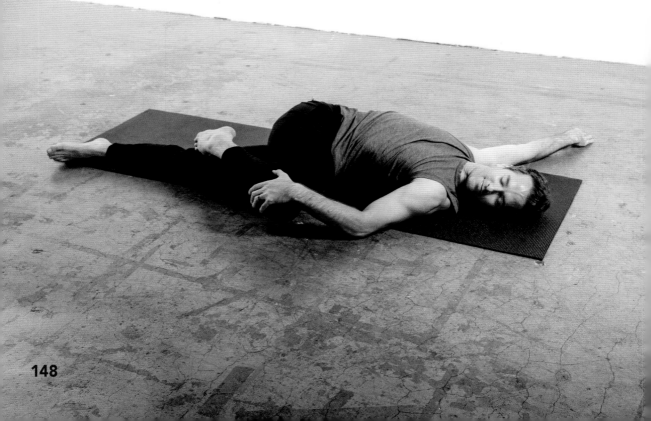

- Place a block or bolster under the bent knee for support.
- Bring both knees into the chest, spread the arms out, and let both knees drape together over to one side (1). For some students, this variation provides a more effective stretch through the lower back.
- Wrap one leg over the top the other and then move into the twist to add more of an outer-hip stretch (2).

MODIFICATION 1

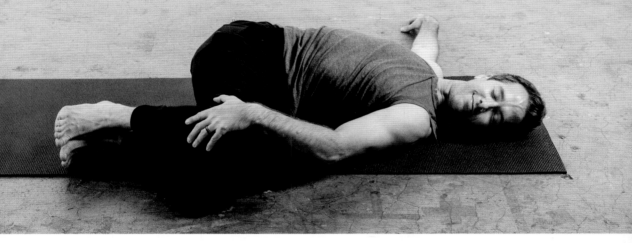

MODIFICATION 2

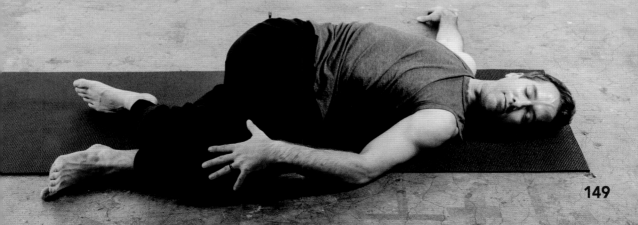

CAT PULLING ITS TAIL POSE

Suggested Duration

2-4 minutes

Benefits

This pose stretches the quadriceps and the chest and massages the spine.

Risks and Contraindications

If you have lower-back pain, proceed carefully.

Alignment Points

- Begin by lying on your back and bring both knees into the belly.
- Extend the right leg out straight and reach the left arm out to the left.
- Allow the left knee to drape across over to the right.
- Rest the right hand on top of the left knee.
- Bend your right knee and reach back with the left hand to grab your right foot.
- Draw your left shoulder blade down into the floor, opening the chest toward the sky.
- Repeat on the other side.

Modifications and Other Options

For a deeper twist, extend the top leg out straight.

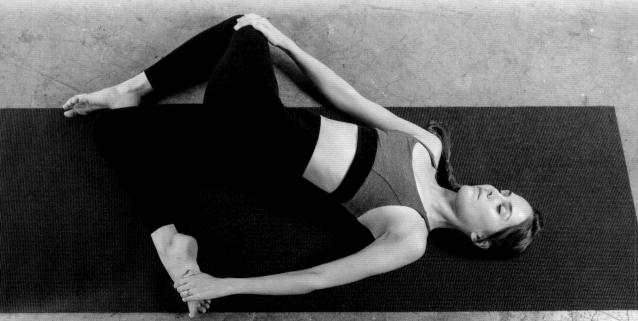

LEGS UP THE WALL

Suggested Duration

5 minutes or more

Benefits

This pose is a cooling, passive alternative to other inversions. It helps drain fluid from the legs, balances hormones, and can reverse the effects of gravity on the body.

Risks and Contraindications

Modify this pose or proceed with caution if you have neck or lower-back pain.

Alignment Points

- While lying on your back, position both legs up the wall toward the ceiling. Slide your sitz bones against to the wall.
- Reach the arms out to the sides or bend the elbows and face the palms toward the ceiling.
- Draw the shoulders down and back and broaden through the chest.

Modifications and Other Options

- If you have a history of neck pain, place a blanket under the head to ensure proper support.
- For additional support for the back, press into the heels, lift the lower back, and slide a bolster or folded blanket under the back. Align the bolster directly under the sacrum, not higher up the back.
- For additional grounding and support, place a light sandbag on the flexed feet.
- Arm variations include bringing the arms into cactus position, with the elbows bent at 90 degrees and the palms facing up, or resting one hand on the belly and the other hand on the chest.

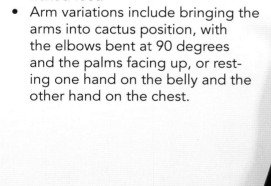

CORPSE POSE

Suggested Duration

5 minutes or more

Benefits

This is the ritual closing pose of any physical yoga practice. It activates the relaxation response and cools the mind. It also helps lower blood pressure.

Risks and Contraindications

Modify this pose if you are pregnant and no longer able to fully recline.

Alignment Points

- Begin on the back with the legs straight out. Allow the feet to relax and fall away from each other.
- Extend the arms by the sides of the body with the palms facing up. Roll the upper arms outward and draw the shoulders down as the shoulder blades move in toward the heart.
- Draw the chin down gently. This will help prevent the head from tilting too far back, which could aggravate the neck.
- Soften the entire body, close the eyes, and rest the body completely.

Modifications and Other Options

- If you are pregnant, use a bolster along the spine for support.
- Students may cover the body with a blanket for warmth or place a folded blanket under the head for support.
- Place a bolster under the knees to help relax the hamstrings and relieve the back muscles.

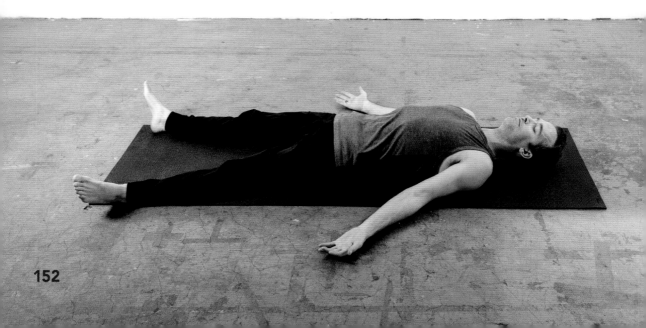

FORWARD NECK STRETCH

Suggested Duration

1-3 minutes

Benefits

This pose releases tension across the back of the neck.

Risks and Contraindications

Proceed carefully if you have neck issues. Exit the pose if you experience sharp pain.

Alignment Points

- Begin in easy seated pose (page 118), sitting up with a tall and straight spine.
- Bring your hands behind your head, interlacing the fingers and letting the elbows flare out.
- Keeping the spine straight, lower the chin toward the chest.
- Let the natural weight of your hands and arms use gravity to produce the stretch without forcing it.

Modifications and Other Options

To target the top of the neck and the base of the skull, gently push the back of your head into your hands.

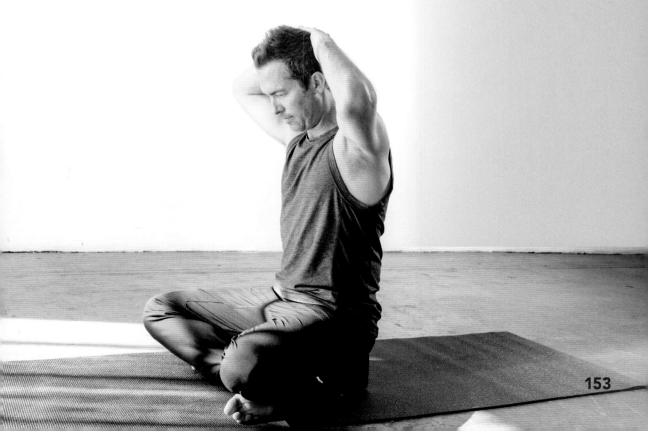

LATERAL NECK STRETCH

Suggested Duration

1-3 minutes

Benefits

This pose allows you to release tension across the entire side of the neck.

Risks and Contraindications

Proceed carefully if you have neck issues.

Alignment Points

- Begin in easy seated pose (page 118), sitting up with a tall and straight spine.
- Reach your left fingertips on the floor away from your hip.
- Take your right hand and place it on the left side of the head.
- Gently release your right ear toward your right shoulder until you feel a stretch across the left side of the neck.
- Repeat on the other side.

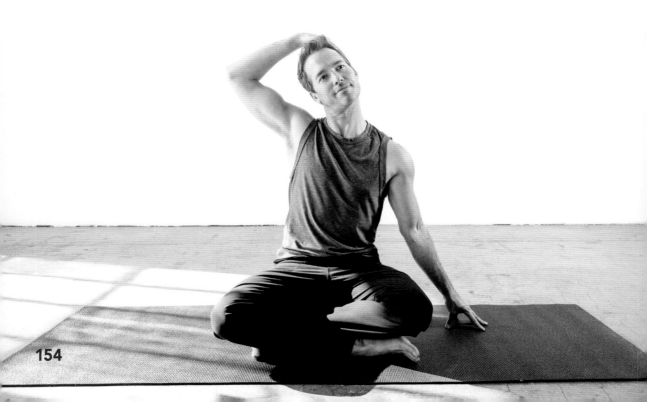

Modifications and Other Options

- For a stretch in the top part of the neck gently release your right ear toward your right shoulder, then turn the chin down toward the right side of the chest until you feel the stretch (1).
- To target the neck muscles at the base of the skull, push the back of the head into your hand to create positive counterresistance (2).

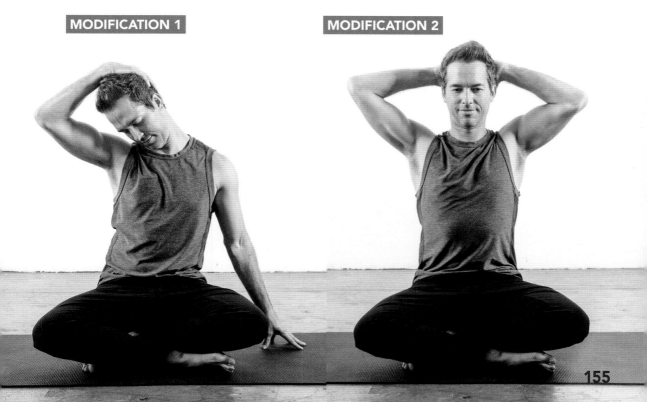

MODIFICATION 1

MODIFICATION 2

155

COW FACE ARMS POSE

Suggested Duration

2-3 minutes

Benefits

This pose provides a great stretch for the shoulders.

Risks and Contraindications

Modify or avoid this pose if you have a shoulder injury.

Alignment Points

- Begin in shoelace pose (page 124) or easy seated pose (page 118).
- Reach your left hand around your back with the palm facing outward.
- Slide your left hand as high up your back as possible. Imagine you are trying to scratch an itch between your shoulder blades.
- Reach your right arm up toward the sky.
- Bending your right elbow, place your right hand behind your neck, with the palm facing inward.
- Bring both hands toward each other until the fingers clasp.
- Repeat on the other side.

Modifications and Other Options

- If your shoulders are tight, use a strap or even a shirt to grab onto. As you hold the stretch, you can work at climbing the hands closer toward each other.
- For a deeper stretch, lean forward.

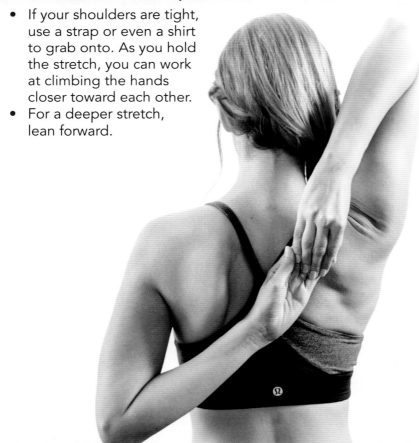

REVERSE PRAYER POSE

Suggested Duration

1-3 minutes

Benefits

This pose provides a deep stretch for the chest, shoulders, wrists, and fore-arms.

Risks and Contraindications

Modify or avoid this pose if you have wrist or shoulder issues.

Alignment Points

- Begin in hero (page 116), shoelace (page 124), or easy seated pose (page 118).
- Bring both hands behind the back and join the palms together with the fingers facing upward.
- Slide the hands as high up the spine as you comfortably can, keeping the palms touching.
- Sit up tall and draw the shoulder blades in toward each other, finding the stretch.
- Keep the chin parallel to the floor.

Modifications and Other Options

- Instead of bringing the palms together, try grabbing el-bows with the opposite hands or making fists and pressing them in toward each other.
- For a deeper stretch, lean forward.

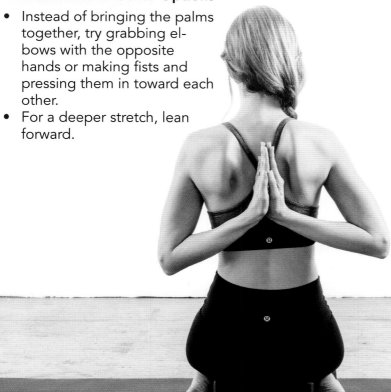

WRIST STRETCH SEQUENCE

Benefits

These stretches promote wrist health and flexibility.

Risks and Contraindications

Students with wrist issues may find these stretches to be too intense. You may not have to go very far to feel the stretch and as long as you are gentle, this sequence should be safe and healing.

Alignment Points

- Begin in saddle pose (page 115) and extend both arms in front of you. Move your hands around in a circular motion eight times one direction and then eight times in the opposite direction (a). Repeat this cycle two more times.
- Come onto all fours. Turn your fingertips outward. Gently sway side to side several times, feeling the stretch in the wrists (b).
- Turn the fingertips back toward the knees and shift backward and forward several times (c and d). Come back, turning the fingertips to face forward for a moment.
- Flip the left hand so that the top of that hand is on the floor with the fingertips facing toward the right knee. Gently pull the hips back toward the heels (e). It doesn't take much movement to feel the stretch. Take several breaths. Then repeat on the other side.

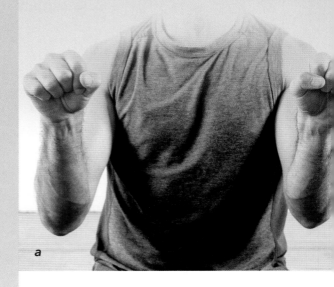

a

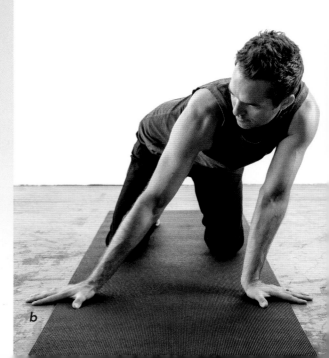

b

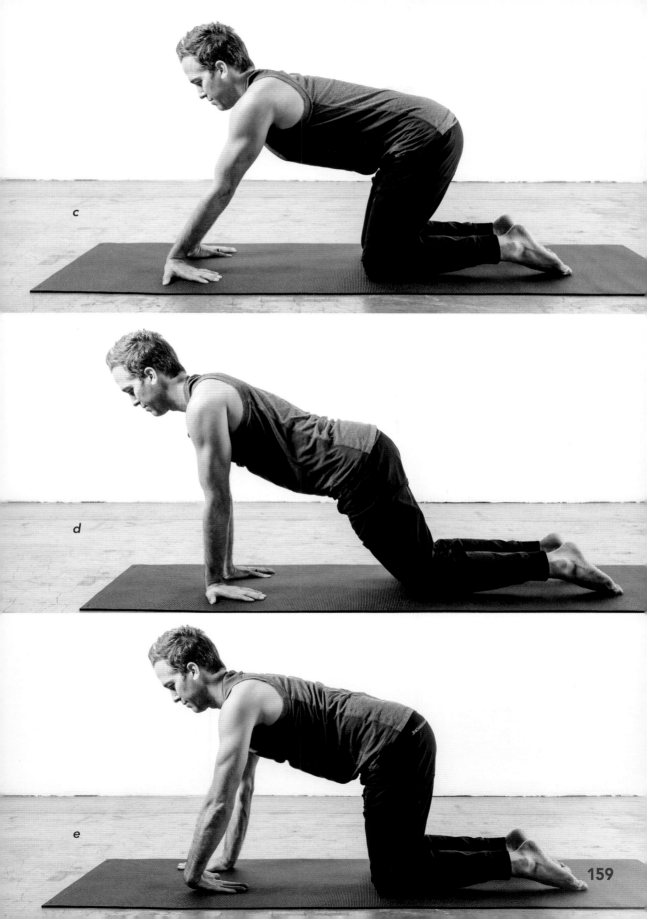

EAGLE ARMS POSE

Suggested Duration

2-3 minutes

Benefits

This pose provides a great stretch for the shoulders, forearms, and wrists and expands the back muscles connected to the shoulder blades.

Risks and Contraindications

Modify or avoid this pose if you have a shoulder injury.

Alignment Points

- Begin in shoelace (page 124), hero (page 116), or easy seated pose (page 118).
- Reach both arms out in front, with your palms facing upward.
- Place the right arm under the left arm and then wrap the forearms around each other until your hands face each other.
- Sit up tall with your chin and biceps parallel to the floor.
- Gently pull your elbows away from the chest, spreading your shoulder blades away from each other.
- Repeat on the other side.

Modifications and Other Options

- Reach both arms in front of you, and bend the left elbow so that the forearm and hand face the sky. Shift the left forearm in front of your face. Reach the right arm over the left arm. Bend the left elbow to deepen the stretch for the outer right shoulder (1). Repeat on the other side.
- For a deeper stretch, lean forward.

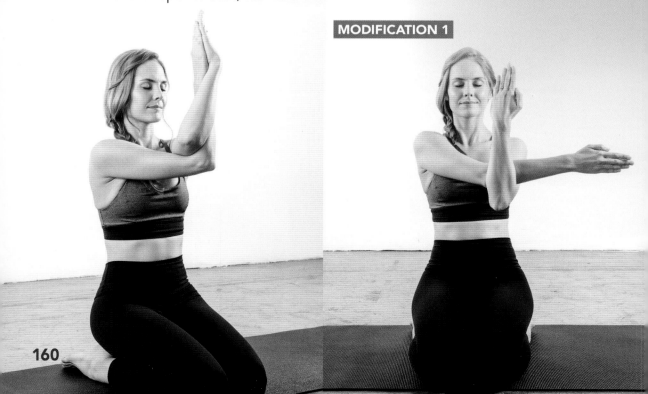

MODIFICATION 1

COUNTERSTRETCHES AND POSES

In yin yoga, we hold the poses a long time, which creates a concentration of chi (life force) in the exposed tissues. After holding a yin yoga pose, it can be beneficial in some cases to move the body to help spread this chi and blood throughout the affected areas. This is done through counterstretches. The counterstretch also provides a powerful release as you move the body in the opposite direction from the yin yoga pose. This allows the tissues an opportunity to rest and reset before moving into the next pose. For example, after holding a long forward bend like half-butterfly pose, the counterstretch half-butterfly backbend moves the torso from flexion into extension, providing a reset for the connective tissues around the spine. The following poses and stretches have a more yang-like quality and are therefore not held as long as the yin poses.

DOWNWARD DOG

Suggested Duration

5-10 breaths

Benefits

This pose is both a strengthening and a rejuvenating posture. It stretches the calf muscles, strengthens the arms and shoulders, and elongates the torso and spine. Downward dog is a great neutralizing pose for the spine when used between a forward bend and a backward bend.

Risks and Contraindications

Modify or avoid this pose if you have serious wrist or shoulder issues.

Alignment Points

- Begin on the hands and knees, tuck the toes, and lift the hips. Place the feet hip-width apart. Spread the toes and align the heels directly behind the second and third toes.
- As the heels descend toward the floor, work the legs toward straight, with the thighs pressing back and the quadriceps engaged. If straightening the legs causes the spine to round, maintain a slight bend in the knees.
- Tilt the sitz bones toward the sky to further lengthen the side of the body and back of the body.
- Place the hands about shoulder-distance apart, with the index fingers pointing straight ahead and the fingers spread wide.
- Straighten the arms and rotate the upper arms outward and slide the shoulders down and back, keeping the neck free and long.
- Align the ears between the upper arms and rest the gaze comfortably.

Modifications and Other Options

- If you have tight hamstrings, spread the feet the width of the mat.
- If your shoulders are tight, rotate your fingers slightly outward.

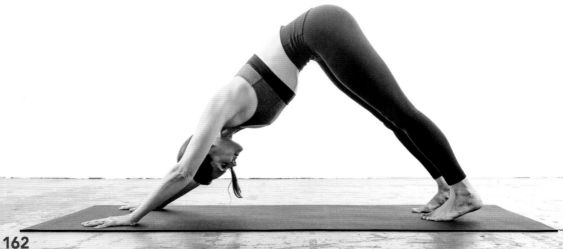

UPWARD TABLE

Suggested Duration

3-5 breaths

Benefits

This pose provides a stretch for the spine, forearms, and wrists. It is a good counterstretch for seated forward-bending poses like caterpillar (page 92) and half-butterfly pose (page 94).

Risks and Contraindications

Modify or avoid this pose if you have serious wrist or shoulder issues.

Alignment Points

- Begin in easy seated pose (page 118), with the hands positioned about 12 inches (30 cm) behind the hips.
- Spread the hands shoulder-width apart, with the fingers facing the back of the mat.
- Position the feet flat on the floor about 12 inches (30 cm) in front of the hips and spread the feet about the width of the shoulders.
- Lean back onto the hands, lift the hips off the ground, and level your belly button with the thighs and the chest.
- Slightly tuck the chin to maintain a long neck.

Modifications and Other Options

- For some students, rotating the fingers forward instead of backward is more comfortable for the wrists and shoulders.
- Turn this movement into a gentle flow by inhaling to lift the hips and exhaling to lower the hips gently to the floor. Repeat for five cycles and hold the last upward table for three to five breaths.

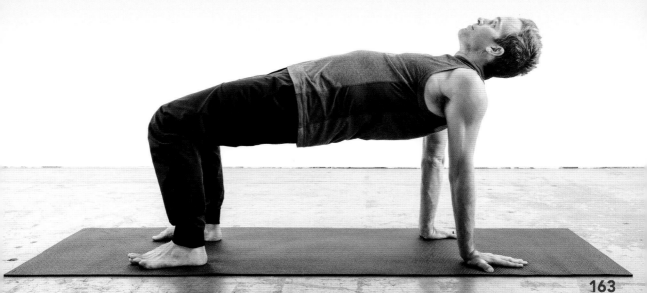

CAT AND COW

Suggested Duration

5-15 cycles

Benefits

This pose stretches both the back and front of the body and stimulates the abdominal organs. This movement is a great counterstretch for both forward and backward bends.

Risks and Contraindications

Keep the neck parallel to the floor if you have a neck injury or pain.

Alignment Points

- Begin on all fours, with the wrists under the shoulders, the knees under the hips, and the tops of the feet flat on the mat.
- Inhale as you drop the belly to the floor and spread across the collar bones (a).
- Exhale as you press into the hands, round through the back, and lift the back of the heart toward the sky (b). Draw the lower belly toward the spine, tuck the tailbone under, and curl the chin in toward the chest.
- Repeat as often as you like, allowing the breath to lead the movement.

Modifications and Other Options

- For a different stretch in the wrist, rotate the fingertips toward the knees.
- Turn this movement into a gentle flow by inhaling while dropping the belly and exhaling while rounding the back.

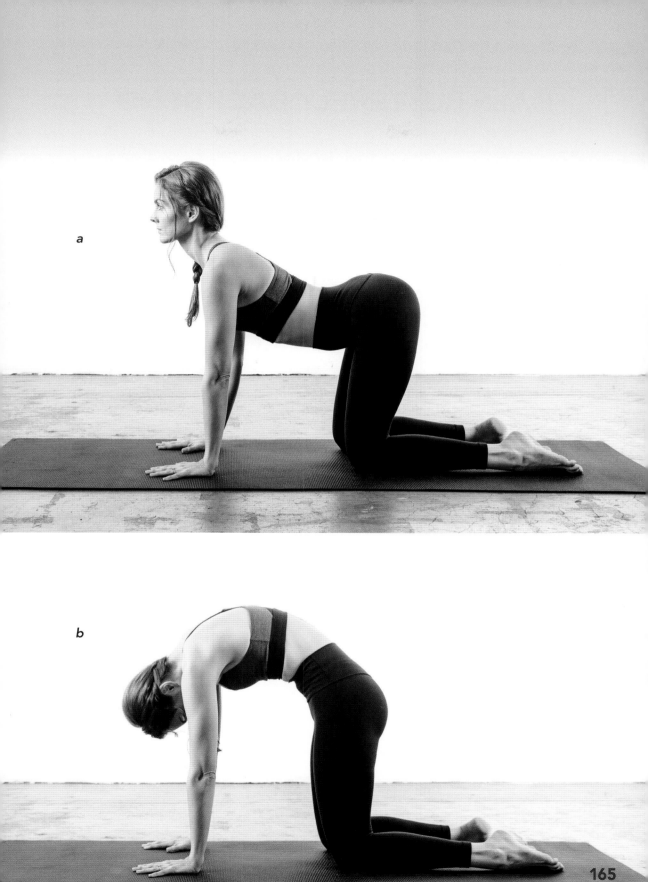

a

b

HALF-BUTTERFLY BACKBEND

Suggested Duration

3-5 breaths

Benefits

This pose stretches the spine and front of the body. It is a great counter-stretch for seated forward bends, especially half-butterfly pose (page 94).

Risks and Contraindications

Proceed with caution if you have wrist pain or spine issues.

Alignment Points

- Begin in a seated position and extend the right leg straight.
- Bend the opposite knee and bring the sole of the left foot into the inner upper thigh of the extended right leg.
- Place the left hand about a foot (30 cm) behind the hips, turning the fingertips away from the body (a).
- Shift the weight into the left hand, lift the hips off the floor, and reach the right arm overhead (b).
- Press the right toes toward the floor.
- Repeat on the other side.

Modifications and Other Options

Turn this movement into a gentle flow by inhaling to lift the hips and exhaling to lower the hips gently to the floor. Repeat for five cycles and hold the last half-butterfly backbend for three to five breaths.

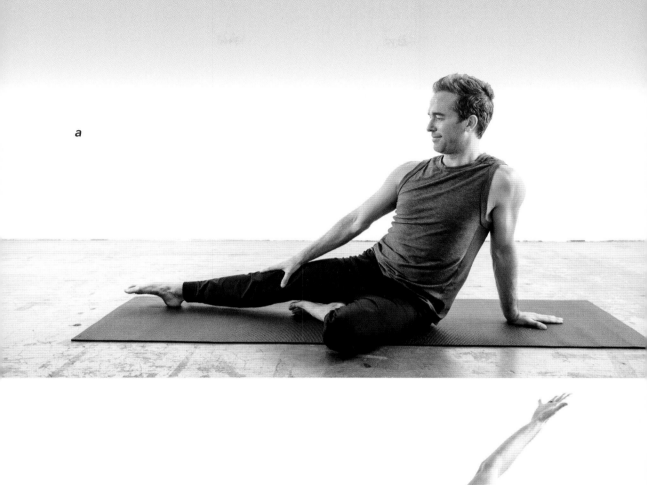

a

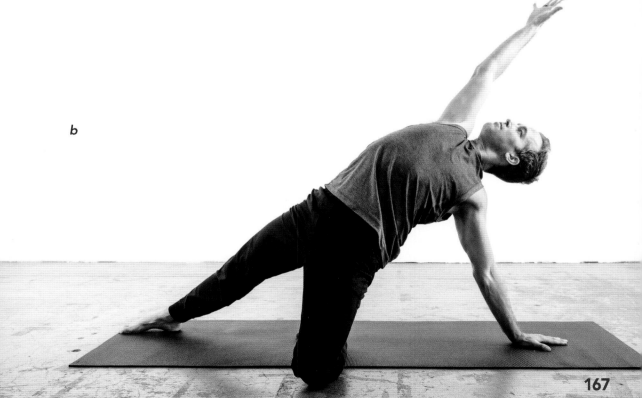

b

HIP CIRCLES

Suggested Duration

5-10 cycles clockwise and 5-10 cycles counterclockwise

Benefits

This movement increases mobility in the hip joints. Secondarily, hip circles stretch the low back, wrists, and shoulders. It is a great counterstretch to poses that stretch the hip, such as sleeping swan (page 123), shoelace (page 124), and fire log (page 126).

Risks and Contraindications

Proceed with caution if you have hip pain.

Alignment Points

- Begin on all fours, with the wrists directly under the shoulders.
- Slide the knees back a few inches behind the hips.
- Circle the entire body around in a clockwise direction (a).
- Circle the entire body around in a counterclockwise direction (b).

Modifications and Other Options

Explore the size of the circles moving from small to larger rotations.

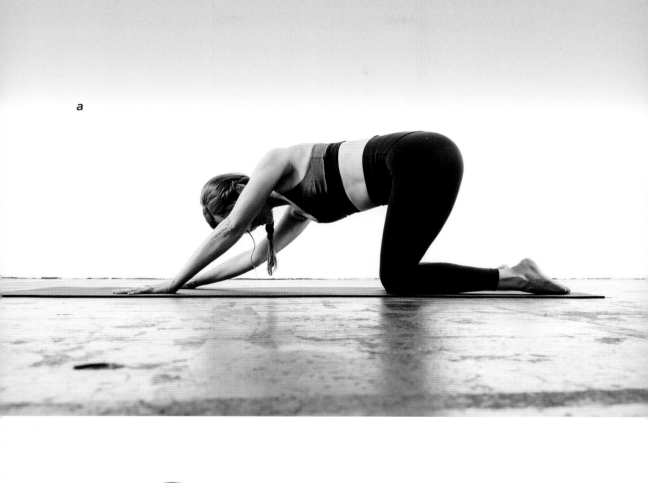

a

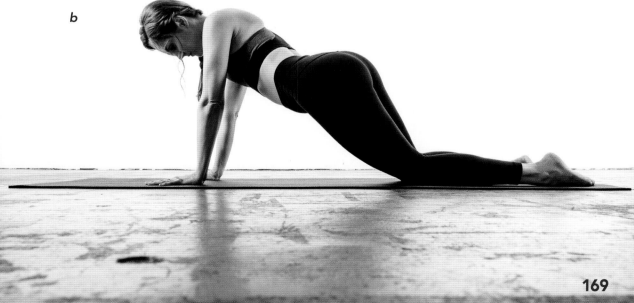

b

WINDSHIELD WIPERS

Suggested Duration

1 minute

Benefits

This movement increases mobility in the hip joints. Secondarily, this pose stretches the ankles, knees, low back, chest, shoulders, and wrists. It is a great counterstretch to poses that stretch the hip, such as sleeping swan (page 123), shoelace (page 124), and fire log (page 126).

Risks and Contraindications

Proceed with caution if you have hip pain.

Alignment Points

- Begin in easy seated pose (page 118).
- Place the hands approximately 12 inches (30 cm) behind the hips.
- Spread the hands shoulder-width apart, with the fingers facing forward.
- Position the feet flat on the floor about 12 inches (30 cm) in front of the hips.
- Spread the feet about the width of the shoulders.
- Gently sway the knees side to side (see a and b).

Modifications and Other Options

As the knees move one direction, turn the gaze in the opposite direction for an added neck stretch.

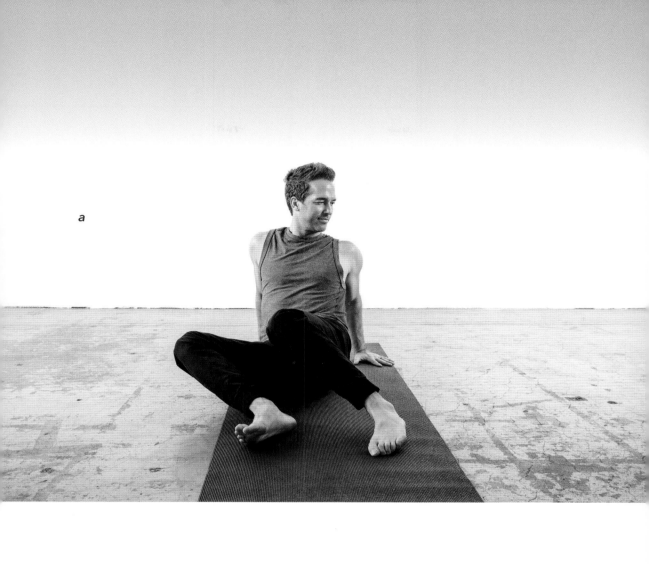

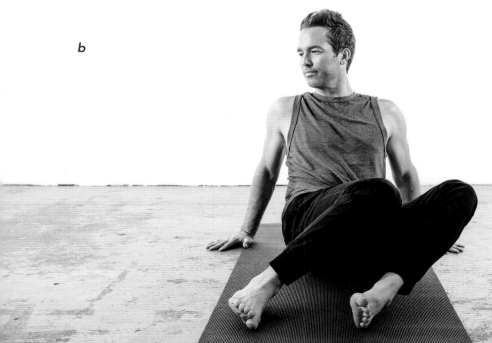

Flo Master

Flo Master has traveled the globe as a featured dancer and personal trainer for singer and songwriter Usher. Flo can commonly be found training with the Ultimate Fighting Championship elite in Redondo Beach, California. His joy, humor, and passion inspires everyone he meets!

T.E. How did you get into yin yoga?

F.M. I had 11 knee surgeries from overtraining and dancing. I was like, "I need to figure out what I'm doing wrong." When Bruce Lee broke his back and the doctor told him he would never walk again, that he'd be paralyzed for the rest of his life, Bruce Lee didn't accept that. He got his ass up. He figured out how to do it, and then he got back up kicking everyone's ass again! [laughter] So I was like, "I got to find that Bruce Lee state of mind. I need to figure out what's going on." So, I stumbled upon yin yoga in *The Ultimate Yogi* program. I was like, "This is what I've been looking for all my life!"

T.E. How did your body feel after doing the yin yoga?

F.M. Having had so many knee surgeries, I was always stiff. I couldn't bend my knees. I couldn't get into positions that I wanted to get into while fighting, dancing, running, and playing. I couldn't do any of that well with my kids. So I started getting into the yin poses and holding the stretches for a long period of time. Everything starts loosening up, and then I could squat more. I could dance longer. I could get out of bed feeling loose. I'm like, "Oh, my God! This is like drugs, right?! This is like drugs to me, like somebody just put some WD-40 into my joints! [laughter] When I don't do yin I'm like the Tin Man from the *Wizard of Oz*. When I do yin yoga, that's like when they put the oil in the Tin Man to make him move. So I was like, "I have to keep up with this."

T.E. Did you ever get Usher to do yin yoga?

F.M. There's a funny story with Usher because he had a bad back, really bad, and he had to perform. I said, "Dude, the problem is you don't stretch." He said, "I stretch a little bit." I'm like, "No. You don't stretch the right way." I said, "You know what? I'm coming out there, I got the perfect guy for you." So, I brought *The Ultimate Yogi* yin yoga DVD up to his hotel. We popped it in, and we did your whole yin yoga. And let me tell you, when he got on stage that night, he was doing stuff that he never thought he could do before! He could literally not stop jumping. I was like, "What the hell is wrong with you?!" He got off stage and he said, "Flo, thank you." And he bought into the yin yoga thing, and he's been doing it ever since.

T.E. That's a great testimonial! Why should an athlete or performer practice yin?

F.M. Nothing is going to work: no squats, no push-ups, no jumps, no pull-ups, no kicking, no punching—none of that means anything if you're tight. Nothing means anything if you don't have mobility or the flexibility in your joints. If you don't stretch, holding the poses for a long period of time to get into the fascia, nothing is going to get better.

T.E. Do you have a favorite yin yoga pose?

F.M. I think my favorite yin yoga pose is probably the sleeping swan. For some reason, it just opens up my hips.

T.E. Do you have a least favorite yin yoga pose?

F.M. The one I try to avoid is reclining half hero. That is the one where I feel like an 85-year-old man!

T.E. Do you have any last "yinspiration"?

F.M. My favorite thing that you say is, "Carrying tension in the body is like driving a car with the emergency brake pulled up." You are going to wear down your pads. So, if you don't stretch, hey, it's your fault!

CHAPTER 6
PRANAYAMA AND MEDITATION

"We can make our mind so like still water that beings gather about us that they may see, it may be, their own images, and so live for a moment with a clearer, perhaps even with a fiercer life because of our quiet."

—William Butler Yeats

In the previous chapter, we learned about yin yoga poses. These poses are healing and beneficial to our physical body, or the annamaya kosha. But what about the deeper layers beyond the physical?

In the beginning of yoga, thousands of years ago, the yogis' primary goal was self-realization and awakening. Like trapped birds being freed from their cages, the yogis dedicated their lives to breaking through the bondages of maya, or the illusion of the material world. When people are stuck in maya, they often live in a state of perpetual suffering. Often, they don't know they are caught in a web of their own misery. This is why awareness is important. It carries people beyond the darkness of ignorance. The yogis viewed this ignorance and suffering as optional. They chose empowerment over victimhood. Through many generations, yogis were able to find a path that gave them freedom and liberation. But it required practices that moved beyond the physical body into the subtle body. Two of these primary practices were pranayama and meditation.

In this chapter, we explore in detail pranayama and meditation and why they are valuable. The physical poses prepare you for these deeper, subtler practices. I've found in my own life that pranayama and meditation are a natural extension of the physical practice. Have you ever tried to sit and consciously breathe or meditate, but you couldn't because of physical discomfort? Perhaps you planned to sit for 30 minutes, but halfway in, your knees started aching, your hips felt stiff, and there was pain in your lower back. Sound familiar? (By the way, these are the primary areas in the body that yin yoga targets!) I know it does for me. And this experience was common for the yogis, too, so they created the poses so they could sit for longer periods without the body getting in the way of their breathing and meditation practices.

Some students may elect to focus only on the physical poses in the beginning and that is perfectly OK. As a teacher, I know this is quite common. However, because the physical practice is limited, eventually the student's growth hits a wall. In the beginning, the physical practice feels exciting, powerful, and transformative. Then one day, you feel like you have stopped growing, and your practice no longer provides what it once did. Typically, at this point, you might start to feel restless, depressed, or no longer motivated and want to quit. This is the point when you should start moving beyond the physical poses into pranayama and meditation.

As you start to challenge yourself in a new way, you will begin to grow again and make all sorts of exciting discoveries. You will find yourself moving into a new chapter of awakening. These awakenings will enhance your physical practice and other aspects of your life. The exciting thing is, there is no limit to the heights you can reach in pranayama and meditation practices. Let's begin by taking a look at the world of pranayama.

PRANAYAMA

Pranayama, the fourth limb of Patanjali's ashtanga yoga, is the science of yogic breathing. The ancient yogis, like the Taoists, studied nature with wonder and passion. They also closely observed and respected the animals within this backdrop of nature. One thing that became apparent to them is that longevity in life is connected to rate of respiration. Animals such as pythons, elephants, and turtles have long lives and their respiration rates are slow. Animals with fast breathing rates, such as birds, dogs, and rabbits, have shorter life spans. A turtle for example, has an average life span of 100 years and breathes approximately 4 breaths per minute. In contrast, a rabbit has an average life span of 10 years and breathes approximately 30-60 breaths per minute. From this observation, yogis surmised that this pattern would transfer to humans. Using themselves as an experiment, they explored slowing their breathing rate. They determined that they could increase their life span through pranayama. Today we know that short, erratic breaths induce stress in the body, exciting the sympathetic branch of the autonomic nervous system. The more stressed the body is, the more quickly the body can break down, which can contribute to disease and impair health and could lead to premature death. In pranayama, the parasympathetic nervous system kicks in, allowing the body to rest and restore. At times, the slower breathing rate can make the heart stronger and better nourished, contributing to a longer and higher quality of life.

Pranayama means the expansion of life force. Prana is the vital energy that is in a constant state of motion, permeating all life and existence. All vibrating energies are prana, including light, heat, electricity, gravity, and magnetism. Pranayama is more than just breath control. It is the technique of expanding the quantity of prana throughout the body. Pranayama must be learned from an experienced teacher only after the student's body and mind have become strong from the practice of the physical postures (asana).

Four Factors of Pranayama

Pranayama requires a mastery of four aspects of the breath. The following are the four factors of pranayama:

- Inhalation (puraka)
- Breath retention after inhalation (antara kumbhaka)
- Exhalation (rechaka)
- Breath retention after exhalation (bahya kumbhaka)

Traditionally, students learning pranayama begin by learning how to exhale properly. Once the exhalation can be performed well, the inhalation will become more powerful. Next, the student moves on to practicing retention after the inhale. After the first three stages are mastered, the student may practice the art of holding the breath at the end of the exhale.

This retention at the end of the exhale is the most difficult part for the average person. It requires letting go. Many people are good at holding on, and the letting go part can be challenging. Physically, the body becomes smaller as we breathe out, and then the retention emphasizes that emptiness. The ego doesn't like to feel empty, small, and insignificant. Often, the resistance that we feel during exhalation and retention is caused by the ego being challenged. This part of the breathing practice has the opportunity to become very transformative. It becomes a practical and visceral way of conquering the ego, which is one of the great themes of yoga and meditation practice.

Anatomy of Breathing

The lungs and diaphragm are located inside the rib cage (see figure 6.1). The diaphragm looks like a jellyfish or the top of a mushroom. The word diaphragm comes from the Greek words for *enclose* and *barricade*. The diaphragm acts as a divider separating the chest and the abdomen. The right half of the diaphragm is slightly higher than the left because of the position of the liver. The

Prana Vayus Within Pranayama

If you recall, in chapter 3, Subtle Anatomy of Yoga, we discussed the prana vayus and that they exist throughout all of nature. They also exist within the four parts of the breath. In fact, each part of the breath is correlated with a season. Inhales are connected to Spring. Breath retention after inhales are connected to Summer. Exhales are connected to Autumn. Retention after exhales are connected to Winter. In this context, you can feel how the rhythm of breath is connected to the rhythm of nature. Let's explore how the prana vayus (page 40) are related to what the chest does during the breathing process:

- Udana vayu: On the inhale, the chest rises.
- Vyana vayu: At the top of the inhale, we hold the breath as the chest expands.
- Apana vayu: On the exhale, the chest lowers.
- Samana vayu: At the bottom of the exhale, we hold the breath as the chest contracts.
- Prana vayu: The cycle of breath continues and we sustain the circle of the breath.

diaphragm moves up and down the torso like a piston inside of a cylinder (figure 6.1*a*). When air flows into the body, the rib cage expands, and the diaphragm moves downward and flattens. This pushes the abdomen out like a balloon (figure 6.1*b*). On exhalation, the diaphragm releases. The abdominal muscles contract and push the air up. As the air leaves the body, the intercostal muscles between the ribs relax and the rib cage becomes smaller (figure 6.1*c*).

When this process is impaired through illness or injury or because a person habitually takes shallow breaths, the function of the diaphragm is limited, leading to short or erratic breathing patterns. This causes the blood to circulate less oxygen through the body and to the brain and activates the sympathetic nervous system, causing the stress reaction of fight or flight. The heart pumps erratically, the mind become anxiety ridden, and the person feels emotionally depleted.

For someone who breathes deeply and rhythmically, the opposite is true. Each breath is full and rich with oxygen. The diaphragm is strong and supple and able to fully function to supply the body with oxygen. The blood vessels of the body and brain dilate, allowing oxygen-rich blood to circulate freely. The parasympathetic nervous system is activated, producing the relaxation response. Natural feel-good chemicals such as endorphins and serotonin are released. The heart pumps steadily, the mind is calm, and the person feels emotionally balanced. I don't know about you, but I'm choosing the second scenario!

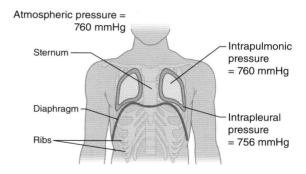

Resting positions of the diaphragm and the thoracic cage, or thorax. Note the size of the rib cage at rest.

a

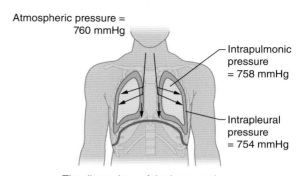

The dimensions of the lungs and the thoracic cage increase during inspiration, forming a negative pressure that draws air into lungs.

b

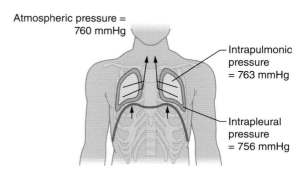

During expiration, the lung volume decreases, thereby forcing air out of the lung.

c

FIGURE 6.1 Lungs and diaphragm *(a)* resting positions, *(b)* inspiration, and *(c)* expiration.

Reprinted by permission from W.L. Kenney, J.H. Wilmore, and D.L. Costill, *Physiology of Sport and Exercise*, 5th ed. (Champaign, IL: Human Kinetics, 2012), 166.

Bandhas Within Pranayama

Although the **bandhas** are not necessary in our yin yoga practice, they can be powerful within our pranayama practice. Bandha means to bind, to hold captive, or to contract. They are locks, or energy seals, that help control, contain, and harness prana, amping up the potency of yoga techniques.

Mula: Root Lock

Mula bandha is activated by contracting the perineum, which causes the pelvic floor to lift. Apana vayu (downward energy) is then rebounded up toward the higher chakras. It produces a purifying heat within the body and rouses the kundalini and helps to control sexual impulses, increases clarity, and decreases the need for food and sleep.

Uddiyana: Abdominal Lock

Uddiyana means to fly up. With this bandha, the abdominal muscles pull up and in, facilitating a natural flow of upward energy. You engage this bandha after mula to help capture the energy and continue to carry it up toward the chest. This powerful bandha strengthens the diaphragm and respiratory muscles, increasing the body's ability to absorb oxygen. It also helps to increase assimilation and elimination within the process of digestion. It is the most powerful of all the bandhas.

Jalandhara: Throat Lock

Jalandhara bandha is engaged by bringing the chin to the chest, causing the throat to contract. It is said to alleviate throat disorders such as inflammation, stuttering, and tonsillitis, and to improve the overall quality of the voice.

I learned the use of bandhas in pranayama from one of my teachers, Srivatsa Ramaswami, who was a long-term student of Krishnamacharya. He taught his students to activate the bandhas during the retention of breath at the end of the exhalation (bahya kumbhaka). The sequence is to first activate mula, then uddiyana, and then jalandhara while holding the breath out. When all three bandhas are engaged simultaneously, they are called the maha bandhas, the great seals. Then, right before taking the next inhalation, release jalandhara, then uddiyana, and then mula. After the retention, the bandhas release, and the next inhalation has greater depth and power. It's almost as if the bandhas create a vacuum effect. During a pranayama practice, this technique causes each cycle of the breath to become more and more powerful.

"It is only by the techniques of pranayama, which regulate, channel, and (in retention of breath) dam the flow all the better to harness and extract its inherent power, that we produce sufficient energy to vitalize the whole system." —B.K.S. Iyengar

Pranayama Postures

Pranayama can be practiced in various positions. Some poses are seated, and some are reclining. Some you feel mostly in the hips, and others you feel more in the knees. Select poses based on your individual needs. Seek a position that sets you up for support and comfort. All poses should create space throughout the torso so there is an abundance of space to breathe into. Listed in each pose are matching pranayama practices.

SUKHASANA:
EASY CROSS-LEGGED
SEATED POSITION

This posture is good for all pranayama practices.

- Come into a comfortable seated position.
- Cross one leg in front of the other.
- Sit up with a tall straight spine.
- Relax the shoulders back and down.
- Allow the outer calves to rest in the inner arches of the feet.
- Rest the hands comfortably on top of the knees.
- You may sit on a prop to elevate the hips for greater comfort.

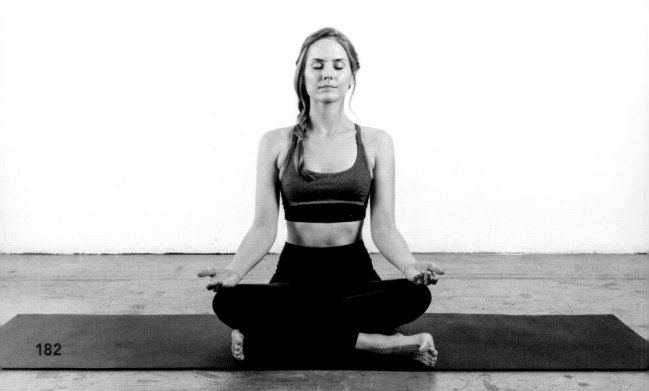

VIRASANA: HERO

This posture is good for all pranayama practices, especially breath of fire (page 193), kapalabhati (page 194), and alternating nostril breathing (page 192).

- Bring the knees together and spread the feet wider than the hips.
- Sit between the feet.
- Sit up with a tall straight spine.
- Relax the shoulders back and down.
- Relax the hands, palms downward on top of the thighs.

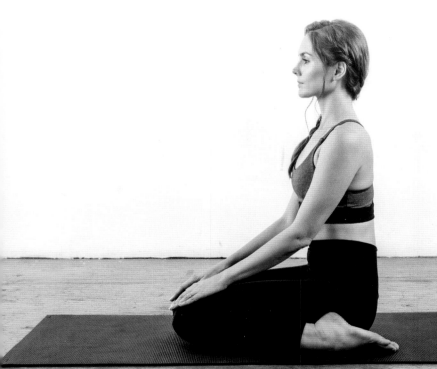

SALAMBA VIRASANA: SUPPORTED HERO

This posture is good for all pranayama practices, especially breath of fire (page 193), kapalabhati (page 194), and alternating nostril breathing (page 192).

- Bring the knees together and spread the feet wider than the hips.
- Sit between the feet on top of a prop.
- Adjust the height of the prop so that the knees are comfortable.
- Sit up with a tall straight spine.
- Relax the shoulders back and down.
- Relax the hands in the lap, or knees, or bring toward the face for alternating nostril breathing.

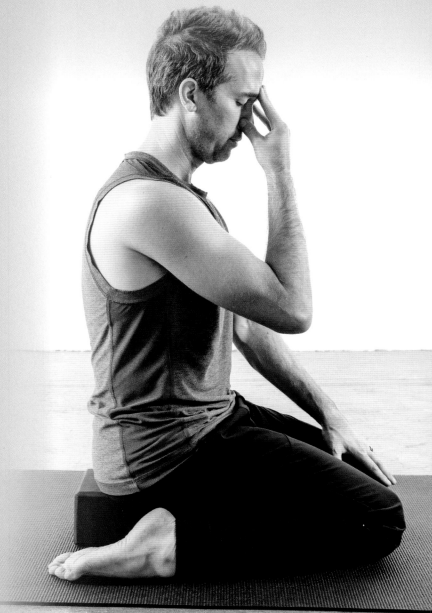

SIDDHASASANA

This posture is good for all pranayama practices.

- Come into a seated position.
- Open the knees wider than sukhasana (page 182).
- Place one foot on top of the other.
- Sit up with a tall straight spine.
- Relax the shoulders back and down.
- Rest the hands of top of the knees.

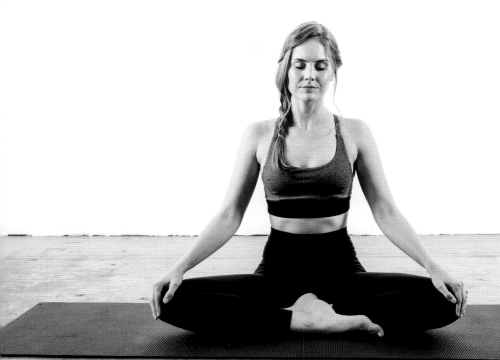

SEATED ON A CHAIR

This posture is good for all pranayama practices, especially ujjayi (page 190) and sama vritti (page 191).

- Sit comfortably toward the middle or front of a chair.
- Place the feet flat on the floor and spread them about shoulder-width apart.
- Sit up with a tall straight spine.
- Relax the shoulders back and down.
- Rest the hands in the lap.

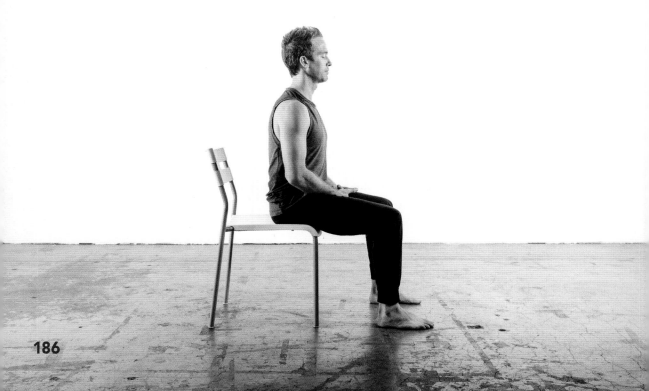

SUPTA BADDHA KONASANA: RECLINING BOUND ANGLE

This posture is good for all pranayama practices except breath of fire (page 193) and kapalabhati (page 194).

- Start by reclining on your back.
- Bring the soles of the feet together with the toes pointing forward and the knees opening outward.
- Either rest the hands next to the body or place one hand on the belly and one hand on the chest.
- You may place props under the knees for support.

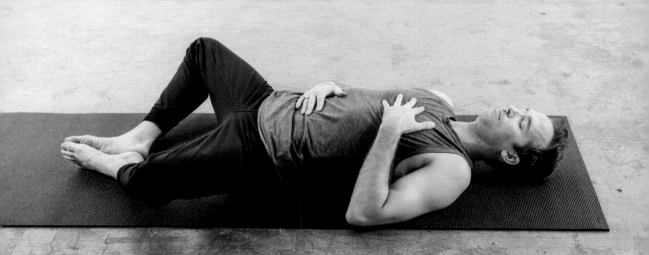

RECLINING TEEPEE

This posture is good for all pranayama practices except breath of fire (page 193) and kapalabhati (page 194).

- Start by reclining on your back.
- Spread the feet about the width of the mat.
- Allow the knees to come together to create support.
- Either rest the hands next to the body or place one hand on the belly and one hand on the chest.

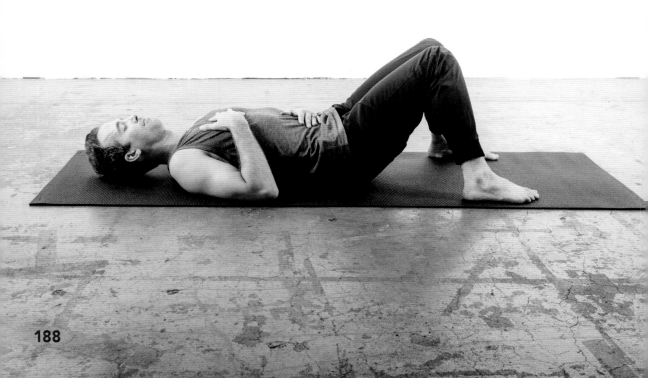

Pranayama Exercises

In this section, we explore different practices of pranayama. You have learned the important context for these ancient breathing practices. Now comes the exciting part where you will understand not just the theory, but also the experience of pranayama. Each practice description will outline how to execute the exercise and list the duration and its benefits. Where it is necessary, appropriate cautions will be given. Before trying the breathing practices, be sure to read the section on practice tips that follows the descriptions.

UJJAYI: VICTORIOUS BREATH

Ujjayi is generated by allowing the flow of breath to pass gently along the glottis, located at the top of the windpipe, creating a soft but audible sound. The sound should be consistent and even on both the inhales and exhales. This sound vibration gives the mind something to sink its teeth into.

Benefits

This is known as the psychic breath because of its effect on the mind. It helps the attention to shift away from the external world of the senses into the internal world of the mind and helps to transcend the force of ignorance.

Exercise

- Inhale for four counts with ujjayi sound.
- Exhale for four counts with ujjayi sound.
- Repeat for 10 rounds.

SAMA VRITTI: EVEN BREATH

Sama means even and *vritti* means wave. This is a great starting pranayama practice that focuses on even inhalations and exhalations. The same amount of energy that is drawn in is then recycled back out.

Benefits

This helps to settle and even the mind through centering and grounding.

Exercise

- Inhale for four counts.
- Hold for four counts.
- Exhale for four counts.
- Hold for four counts.
- Repeat for 10 rounds.

NADI SHODHANA: ALTERNATING NOSTRIL BREATHING

Nadi means pathway or channel. **Shodhana** means cleansing. Nadi shodhana helps to purify the right and left channels of the body, bringing them into balance. Because nadi shodhana balances both hemispheres of the brain, it is a powerful pranayama.

Benefits

This breathing technique calms and centers the mind and brings it back to the present. It works therapeutically for most circulatory and respiratory problems and maintains body temperature. It also releases accumulated stress, balances the logical and emotional sides of our personalities, and contributes to an overall flow of prana throughout the body.

Exercise

- Start by emptying the lungs on an exhale. Close the right nostril with the right thumb. Inhale through the left nostril for four counts, and then hold for two counts.
- Seal the left nostril with the right ring finger and exhale through the right nostril for four counts, and then hold for two counts.
- Inhale through the right nostril for four counts, and then hold for two counts.
- Seal the right nostril with the right thumb and exhale through the left nostril for four counts, and then hold for two counts.
- Repeat the cycle eight times.

BHASTRIKA: BREATH OF FIRE

This is a powerful pranayama for opening the pranavaha srotas (respiratory channels), giving equal emphasis on both the inhalations and exhalations as you pump air in and out through the nose. The focus of attention should be on the chest and lungs. Throughout the practice, the body should remain steady, especially the shoulders and chest. Only the lungs, diaphragm, and abdomen should move. The face should be as relaxed as possible: in other words, no scary Halloween faces!

Benefits

Breath of fire strengthens the diaphragm and stimulates the heart, increasing blood circulation. It massages the brain and stimulates the circulation of cerebral fluid. The powerful pumping of the breath purifies cells by washing out stagnant waste gases. It helps to clear away mucus in the sinuses and builds up greater resistance against colds and other respiratory disorders. It improves digestion and accelerates metabolic activity. Regular practice of breath of fire strengthens the nervous system.

Exercise

- For 60 seconds, breathe rapidly in and out through the nose and allow the belly to pump in and out.
- Emphasize both inhalation and exhalation.
- Bring your awareness to the chest and lungs.
- If you feel overly dizzy, slow down and allow the pumping of the breath to soften.

KAPALABHATI: SKULL SHINING BREATH

Similar to breath of fire, kapalabhati is considered to be a kriya (cleansing exercise), but it is often used in pranayama practice. When I studied pranayama in depth with my teacher Srivatsa Ramaswami, we commonly started with this practice before transitioning into others. For this exercise, breathe in and out through the nose, emphasizing the exhalations by imagining a blacksmith's bellows forcefully pumping the air out. The primary focus should be on the nasal cavity, and the breaths should be almost like simulated sneezes. This practice is said to be the destroyer of all mucous disorders. Also, it activates the pituitary and pineal glands by invigorating the brain.

Benefits

Kapalabhati massages the brain by compressing and decompressing the cerebrospinal fluid. It purifies the cells and lungs by expelling waste gases. The vitality of the cells is animated as the blood is saturated with an abundance of oxygen. It raises the alkalinity of the blood chemistry by releasing carbon dioxide out of the body. It keeps the spongy tissue of the lungs supple. Similar to breath of fire, it cleans the sinuses and respiratory passages. It tones the abdominal organs and massages the diaphragm and liver. Skull shining breath invigorates the brain and awakens subtle perception.

Exercise

- Pump air in and out through the nose, emphasizing the exhalations. The inhalations should be a natural reflex.
- Focus your attention on your nose and nasal passages.
- Perform one round of 36 kapalabhati repetitions, and then take five ujjayi recovery breaths.
- Repeat this cycle twice more for a total of 108 kapalabhati repetitions.
- If you experience dizziness, slow down and soften the kapalabhati repetitions.

VILOMA I: INTERRUPTED INHALATIONS

Vi means negation or against. *Loma* means hair or grain. So, viloma means against the grain. This pranayama pauses ujjayi breath on the inhale once or twice.

Benefits

This heightens breath awareness and improves breath control. It also emphasizes the power of taking in or receiving.

Exercise

- Inhale for two counts.
- Pause for two counts.
- Inhale for two more counts to the top of the lungs.
- Exhale for four counts, emptying the lungs.
- Repeat for 10 rounds, activating the ujjayi breath.

VILOMA II: INTERRUPTED EXHALATIONS

Vi means negation or against. *Loma* means hair or grain. Viloma means against the grain. This pranayama pauses ujjayi breath on the exhale once or twice.

Benefits

This heightens breath awareness and improves breath control. It also emphasizes the power of release and letting go.

Exercise

- Inhale for four counts.
- Exhale for two counts.
- Pause for two counts.
- Exhale for two more counts, emptying the lungs.
- Repeat for 10 rounds, activating the ujjayi breath.

VISHAMA VRITTI: UNEQUAL RATIO

Vishama means uneven, irregular, or dissimilar. In this unequal ratio pranayama, the duration of inhalations and exhalations is different. One of the versions of this exercise most favored by yogis is using a ratio of one count of inhalation for every two counts of exhalation.

Benefits

This pacifies the brain and nervous system and strengthens the ability to detach and let go in a positive way.

Exercise

- Inhale for four counts.
- Hold for four counts.
- Exhale for eight counts.
- Hold for four counts.
- Repeat for 10 cycles.

The Three Primary Nadis

The nadis are fine, wirelike channels that run throughout the body, transferring the flow of prana. Just like excess fats can accumulate in the blood vessels and block the flow of blood, a buildup of waste in the nadis can block the flow of prana. These blockages inhibit the natural movement of energy. Energy decreases, and the body becomes lethargic. Activation of the higher brain and chakras is impeded. Exercising the body with mindfulness, eating wholesome food, and pranayama practice ensure that the nadis remain open and pure.

Classic yoga texts offer several perspectives on the number of nadis, but they all cite thousands and thousands of channels. Although there are thousands of nadis, the three most important are the sushumna, ida, and pingala.

- The sushumna nadi originates at the base of the spine in the tailbone. It moves up to the crown of the head. Within this central channel are located the seven chakras.
- The pingala nadi starts at the base of the spine and spirals up to the right nostril. The pingala is aligned with yang energy, representing a strong, masculine, and solar energy. It is also related to the sympathetic nervous system. Right-nostril breathing is linked to the left hemisphere of the brain, the analytical, logical, and reasoning part of the brain.
- The ida nadi starts at the base of the spine and spirals up to the left nostril. The ida is aligned with yin energy, representing a receptive, feminine, and lunar energy. It is associated with the parasympathetic nervous system. Left-nostril breathing is linked to the right hemisphere of the brain, the creative, imaginative, and intuitive part of the brain.

Although the benefits of pranayama practice are powerful, it is imperative that you progress slowly and steadily. In our culture, we often want things to come fast and furiously. Think about your pranayama practice like a marathon instead of a sprint. Move forward with the wisdom of patience.

Just to be clear, I cannot overemphasize the importance of working with prana respectfully. Imagine that your nervous system is like a circuit board. If you run too much voltage of electricity through the board, then you will blow a fuse and cause permanent damage. The human body is the same. This is why Patanjali, in the *Eight Limbs of Yoga*, put the physical poses before the practice of pranayama. The yoga poses create a strength and stability within the human body that can effectively harness an increase of life force that pranayama practice invokes. If one jumps into pranayama prematurely or moves too fast, then nervous system issues such as shakiness, tremors, anxiety, and depression can arise. I've met and received correspondence from concerned people that this has happened to. Recently, a student who was in my pranayama and meditation training shared with the group about a time when she suffered from a seizure while doing pranayama with an inexperienced teacher. She was traumatized from the experience, but fortunately, our time together initiated her healing process.

I don't want to scare you, but take your time to progress slowly and carefully as the practices have been outlined in this chapter. Have respect for the awakening of prana within the body. Think of prana like a cobra and you are a cobra trainer. An unskilled trainer can be bitten, but the skilled trainer harnesses the energy of the cobra. Be skillful and enjoy all the clarity, energy, and power that the practices of pranayama provide.

Pranayama Practice Tips

Pranayama is typically sequenced after the physical practice and before meditation. Your pranayama practice should take place in a quiet and clean space with minimal clutter. The space should be well ventilated to prevent breathing in harmful particles. The temperature of the space should be slightly warm, but avoid practicing in direct sunlight unless it is sunrise or sunset. Also, avoid heavy drafts or an overhead fan that can disrupt the element of air within the body. If cold weather or insects are an issue, cover your body with a sheet or blanket for protection.

Although the best time to practice pranayama is in the early morning, find the time that works best for you. As much as possible, try to practice at the same time and in the same place each day. No matter what time of day you practice pranayama, be sure that it's done on an empty stomach. Generally, it is good to wait three to four hours after eating a meal because food in the stomach will inhibit full respiration from taking place and can cause nausea during some of the deeper pranayama practices. Choose a duration that works for your schedule. This could be 5 minutes or 45 minutes. The key is regularity.

Use deeper and more invigorating pranayamas in the morning. This might include breath of fire (bhastrika) and skull shining breath (kapalabhati). You can use more soothing and relaxing pranayamas in the evening before bed. This could include even breath (sama vritti), alternating nostril (nadi shodhana), or unequal ratio (vishama vritti). No matter which pranayama you use, the key is to avoid strain while practicing because much of the power of pranayama comes through allowing as opposed to striving. Through a regular and steady practice, you will feel over time an increase in prana. All the benefits will come to you naturally.

MEDITATION

If I told you that I had a pill that would boost your immunity, improve memory, lower blood pressure, increase clarity and creativity, decrease stress hormones, improve digestion, reduce wrinkles, give you better skin, decrease suffering, and improve your happiness, I bet you would be willing to pay big bucks for that. Right? Well, that magic pill exists and it's called *meditation*.

> *"Between stimulus and response there is a space.*
> *In that space is our power to choose our response.*
> *In our response lies our growth and our freedom."*
> *—Viktor E. Frankl*

Meditation is yoga that takes place inside the mind. In meditation, we take time out of our busy schedules to become quiet and go within, to deepen our relationship with ourselves and become the observer of our own thoughts. Inevitably, our thoughts lead to actions, our actions lead to habits, our habits lead to our personality, and our personality leads to our present reality. Simply put, everything traces back to the thoughts moving through your mind. To shift your outer reality, you must start by shifting what's happening within.

The real battle is the one that takes place inside the mind. During meditation, if you experience boredom or resistance, or if the ego rears its ugly head, screaming, "Stop! You're wasting your time," just know that you are not alone. In fact, one particular Tibetan lama describes the process of meditation as being "one insult after another!" This is why so many people talk about meditation but don't practice it. It's difficult to erase old mental programs we've established, but if you conquer your mind, you will start to establish mental programs that are conducive to living the kind of life you want to live.

When meditation is practiced regularly, the benefits are plentiful. Here is just a sample of the beneficial effects:

Boosts immune system

Improves memory

Increases sex hormones

Lowers blood pressure

Increases clarity

Increases creativity

Decreases stress hormones

Restores the body even more than sleep does

Increases gray matter in the brain

Bridges the left and right hemispheres of the brain

Increases happiness

"Our true home is the present moment."
—Thich Nhat Hanh

Meditation Postures

In meditation, there are four main postures (see figure 6.2). No matter what your body type is, one of the positions will work for you. You might have a favorite position, but periodically your physical needs change, so you should alter your posture accordingly. For example, I've had students who have gone through cancer treatment, and asking them to meditate in any position besides reclining would be unrealistic. Also, sometimes you have to adjust to the environment you are in, such as your office, in-law's house, car, or an airport. The four meditation postures are cushion (6.2*a*), chair (6.2*b*), reclining (6.2*c*), and walking (6.2*d*).

Meditation Practices

Many schools of meditation exist. The following are eight powerful practices that are appropriate for all levels. If you are new to meditation, I recommend trying each one. After exploring them all, you can choose the one that resonates with you the most. Once you select your practice, stick to it for minimum of 28 days. This is important because anything you repeat will change over time. In the beginning, you might have a lot of exciting and pleasurable experiences. Then down the road, boredom and challenges might arise. It is at this point that the magic starts to happen. If you switch meditation practices prematurely, you will miss an opportunity for deeper transformation. When digging a well, you don't want to dig a bunch of shallow holes; you want to dig one deep hole that taps into the underground water. In the case of meditation practice, the underground water is your true nature. Take your time selecting a meditation practice that resonates with you, and as mentioned previously, stay with it for a minimum of 28 days.

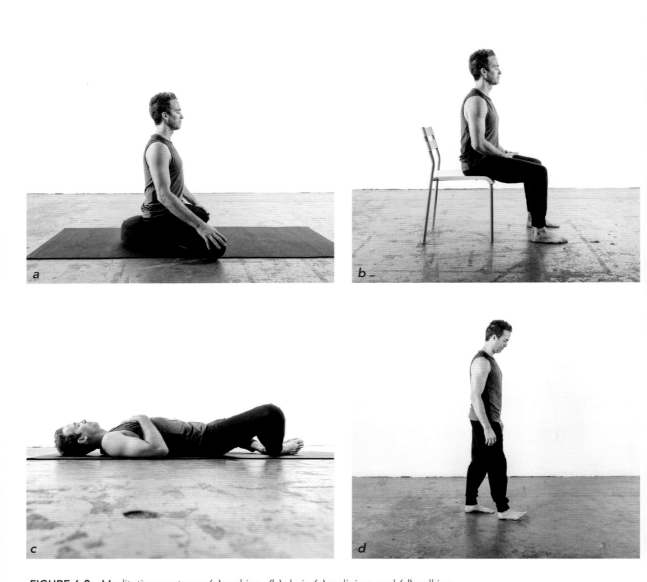

FIGURE 6.2 Meditation postures: (a) cushion, (b) chair, (c) reclining, and (d) walking.

Gratitude Meditation

Gratitude is a high-vibrational place. Begin to focus on all the things you are grateful for. Feel a surge of gratitude swelling within as you give thanks for the blessings that exist in your life, such as your home, access to food, clothes, the planet, the beautiful places you've experienced, the amazing people in your life, and, most important, the miracle of you. What you give gratitude toward, you attract more of into your life.

Dedication Meditation

Summon within your heart a person or place facing significant challenges—a person battling a life-threatening disease, a region of the planet going through a war, a place that has experienced a natural catastrophe, or even a family pet struggling with an illness. Visualize the object of your dedication being showered and bathed with good vibes. Maybe repeat a prayer several times. This is a form of karma yoga, the yoga of selfless action, and you can be assured that your subject will benefit from your thoughts and prayers.

Bring-Your-Own-Mantra Meditation

The things you think are the things you become. Choose a quality that you would like to strengthen within yourself. It could be forgiveness, compassion, creativity, health, or love, so long as it has resonance for you. Once you've chosen your quality, plug it into the sentence, "I am _____." So, if you selected health, it would be "I am health." Now, internally recite the quality over and over, keeping the mind focused on the mantra.

Repetition Meditation

Repetition meditation is similar to BYOM meditation, except that you repeat the chosen quality by itself, stripping away the words "I am." For example, "Health. Health. Health." Each time you repeat the quality, you are driving it deeper into the soil of your consciousness. Imagine every cell in your body illuminated as the total embodiment of your chosen quality.

So Hum Meditation

This meditation is over 3,000 years old. A simple but powerful technique, *so hum* meditation uses the breath and the repetition of a mantra to quiet the mind and relax the body. This meditation will help take your awareness from a state of constriction to a state of expanded consciousness. On an inhale, gently and internally say the word *so*. On an exhale, gently and internally say the word *hum*. Notice how the word *so* reflects the sound of the inhalation and how the word *hum* reflects the sound of the exhalation. Let your breath remain natural as you repeat the mantra, bringing your awareness back to it each time the mind becomes distracted by a thought, sound, or sensation. Let the mantra align with the breath, and between breaths, allow your awareness to rest in the spaces between the cycles.

Vedic-Style Meditation

In the Vedic style of meditation, the mind is focused on a simple mantra. In this meditation, use the mantra *ram*, which represents goodness, strength, and truth. Internally, repeat the mantra in a gentle manner. When the mind wanders, let the distraction go and come back to repeating the mantra. Over time, you can slow the repetition so there are longer spaces of stillness between the mantra.

Loving-Kindness Meditation

Metta is the Pali word for loving kindness. Pali was the language spoken in India during the time of the Buddha. In this traditional metta meditation, loving-kindness is directed toward different categories of people. Metta meditation does not depend on whether one deserves loving-kindness or not, it is not restricted to friends and family, and it extends out from personal connections to include all beings. The meditation begins with loving ourselves, because unless we have love for ourselves, it is difficult to extend it to others. Eventually, we expand beyond ourselves to include others who are special to us and then to the whole planet. Throughout the meditation, repeat the following three phrases:

May you be safe.

May you be happy.

May you be at peace.

Call yourself to mind. See yourself as you are today or visualize yourself as a young child. As you hold yourself compassionately, send the phrases of loving kindness to yourself.

Next, call to mind a benefactor or someone who supported you. This could be a teacher, mentor, family member, friend, or spiritual guide. See this person clearly in your mind and send them the phrases.

Third, bring to mind someone you love and care for. See this person clearly in your mind and send them the phrases.

Fourth, bring to mind a neutral person. This is someone you can see clearly in your mind, but whom you do not have strong feelings of like or dislike for. This might be someone you see at the grocery store, in your neighborhood, or at your local coffee shop. You might not know their name or know anything about them. See them clearly and send them the phrases.

Finally, bring to mind all beings everywhere. Visualize the world, your local community, people both near and far, all animals and plants. Send all beings everywhere the phrases of loving kindness.

At the end of your meditation, sit in complete stillness and silence. Finish by feeling light, which is the key word in enlightenment. Slowly open your eyes, bringing serenity with you, as you shift from the internal world back to the external world.

Chakra Meditation

As we explored in depth in chapter 3, the chakras are the primary energy centers that run along the central corridor inside the spine. These energy centers are connected to various elements, colors, mantras, and subtle qualities. The following meditation is a way to purify and activate each of the seven chakras. When repeating the affirmations and mantras, you can do so either silently or out loud.

Finding a comfortable seated position, sit up tall and close your eyes, relax your shoulders, and soften your face. Begin by taking a few steady breaths in and out through the nose.

Bring your attention down into the tailbone, or the base of the spine, connecting to the muladhara chakra. Keeping your attention in this place, visualize the color red, and feel a connection to the element of earth. Repeat the following affirmation, "I am grounded and steady." After a short pause, repeat the bija mantra *lam* three times. Take a few moments to imagine the muladhara chakra spinning in a balanced, steady way.

Shift your attention up to the sacrum and pelvic basin, connecting to the swadhisthana chakra. Holding your attention in this place, visualize the color orange, and feel a connection to the element of water. Repeat the following affirmation, "I am creative and fluid." After a short pause, repeat the bija mantra *vam* three times. Take a few moments to imagine the swadhisthana chakra spinning in a balanced, steady way.

Bring your attention to the upper abdominals, or the solar plexus region, connecting to the manipura chakra. Holding your attention in this place, visualize the color yellow, and feel a connection to the element of fire. Repeat the following affirmation, "I am strong and powerful." After a short pause, repeat the bija mantra *ram* three times. Take a few moments to imagine the manipura chakra spinning in a balanced, steady way.

Shift your attention up to the middle of the chest, connecting to the anahata chakra. Holding your attention in this place, visualize the color green, and feel a connection to the element of air. Repeat the following affirmation, "I am generous and kind." After a short pause, repeat the bija mantra *yam* three times. Take a few moments to imagine the anahata chakra spinning in a balanced, steady way.

Bring your attention to the center of the throat, connecting to the vishuddha chakra. Holding your attention in this place, visualize the color blue, and feel a connection to the element of air. Repeat the following affirmation, "May my words and speech uplift and inspire." After a short pause, repeat the bija mantra *hum* three times. Take a few moments to imagine the vishuddha chakra spinning in a balanced, steady way.

Shift your focus up to the center of the forehead, connecting to the ajna chakra. Holding your attention in this place, visualize the color purple, and feel a connection to the element of space. Repeat the following affirmation, "I am guided by wisdom and intuition." After a short pause, repeat the bija mantra *om* three times. Take a few moments to imagine the ajna chakra spinning in a balanced, steady way.

Last, bring your awareness to the crown of the head, connecting to the sahasrara chakra. Holding your attention there, visualize a white light emanating from the top of the head. Feel yourself transcending all the elements. Repeat the following affirmation, "I am connected to my higher power." After a short pause, sit in the power of silence and stillness. Pause, and then finish by taking a few minutes to imagine all seven chakras spinning in a balanced, steady way. Slowly, open the eyes.

Common Excuses for Not Meditating

Many people know and understand the great benefits of meditation but still resist it. Perhaps you have resisted starting, or you have tried to meditate, but failed to lock it into a regular habit. These obstacles are quite normal. In fact, anything worthwhile in life is going to involve struggle and challenge. By being committed and overcoming these challenges, you will grow mentally and emotionally. Let's look at the most common excuses people give for not meditating.

"I don't have time."

You have to take time in order to make time. Meditation practice makes you more efficient and more effective. Mistakes and accidents are greatly reduced when you take the time to pause and center yourself. If you do so, chances are you will be able to maintain your sense of inner calmness when you find yourself in an environment where you must be highly productive. This is the power of presence. With all the time that people spend on social media or watching television, you can definitely carve out a little time for your meditation practice. It's about managing your time well. Many of the most successful CEOs, filmmakers, athletes, and entertainers practice meditation. Despite demanding schedules, they find time to meditate, even on the busiest and most stressful days. If they can do it, you can do it.

"I don't know where to start."

Start simple and small. At the end of this chapter are eight powerful meditations. If you can carve out just five minutes, then start there. Like everything else, the key is consistency. As world-renowned motivational speaker and author Tony Robbins says, "Repetition is the mother of skill." The benefits will come from getting on your meditation cushion every day. There are also lots of great meditation apps you can download onto your smartphone.

"When I meditate nothing happens, and I can't stop my thoughts."

Just as the salivary glands secrete saliva, the mind secretes thoughts. This is a natural process. Instead of stopping your thoughts, allow yourself to direct them. Many people have the misconception that when they meditate, they are supposed to feel blissful and experience an endless state of rapture. Although this is possible, the point in meditation is to be with whatever is naturally there. Your meditation practice is like a mirror: It will reflect back to you whatever is currently happening for you. If you are agitated, then it will reflect agitation. If you are joyful, then it will reflect joy. The point is to not judge, resist, or push away what is revealed to you. By watching and observing your natural state, you will access a part of you that is bigger and more spacious than the thought or feeling. From this place, you will find yourself less entangled and more free.

"When the power of love overcomes the love of power, the world will know peace." —Jimi Hendrix

Meditation Practice Tips

To start, find a quiet, clean, comfortable place in your home devoted solely to your meditation practice. It can be a room or even just a corner, but this will be your spot for finding stillness. For some people, practicing at home may not be possible. Other options are finding a place at work or even meditating in your car. (Just make sure you are not driving and meditating at the same time!) Select a time when you will be uninterrupted. For many of us, early in the morning is ideal, but find the time that works for you.

Once you have found your meditation posture, keep a few things in mind. Each of the following suggestions will provide greater clarity for your practice, which is especially helpful for beginners. The more you practice these simple tips, the more natural and effortless they will feel. Eventually they will become second nature.

Spine, Head, and Neck

Keep the chin parallel to the floor. You can even tilt the chin slightly down, creating more length and space in the neck. Keep the spine tall in a relaxed and noble manner. Some students benefit from supporting their back by sitting in a chair or against a wall. In certain situations, reclining may be necessary. In this case, placing a pillow under the knees and padding under the head or neck can be helpful. Just like when you are seated, keep the neck open by leveling the forehead with the chin. In most situations, it is advisable to choose seated over reclining. In meditation, we want to remain awake and alert. Reclining onto the floor can often make you drowsy and sleepy.

Gaze

In meditation, we often close the eyes. If sleepiness or past trauma is an issue, then the eyes may stay open. In this situation, you want to relax and soften the gaze. Look at a single, unmoving point and proceed with the meditation practice.

Arms and Hands

When seated, allow the hands to rest comfortably in the lap or on top of the thighs. Allow the shoulders to relax and the elbows to have a comfortable bend. Typically, the palms face up, with the intention of allowing and receiving. In certain situations, turning the palms downward can invoke an energy of grounding. When reclining, the arms can rest effortlessly along the body, or the hands may be placed wherever it feels right.

Feet and Legs

When seated on the floor, it is helpful to elevate the hips higher than the knees by sitting on a cushion or prop. This can minimize discomfort in the knees. Placing props under the knees can minimize discomfort in the hips. These supports become beneficial in longer meditation sits. When seated in a chair, allow both feet to rest flat on the floor. Position the feet about hip-width apart, finding comfort and stability. In the event that the feet do not reach the floor, place something firm under the feet.

Stillness

In meditation practice, just like in yin yoga, stillness is important. You want to become as still as possible, minimizing fidgeting. For new meditators, it is common for distracting sensations to arise. You might feel an itch here, an itch there, and then some sort of uncomfortable sensation somewhere else. Then you unconsciously react to those sensations, which keeps you stuck within habitual patterns. Before reacting to a sensation, observe it. In many cases it will pass or change in some way. If the sensation persists and causes moderate discomfort, feel free to adjust the body. The key is to adjust and move mindfully.

In this chapter, we investigated the power of pranayama and meditation. These practices are sure to complement and expand your yin yoga practice to the next level. Come back to this chapter numerous times to explore the different varieties of practice. The next chapter is about empowering yourself. You will build on everything you have learned and dive into developing a personal practice.

Matt Kahrs

Matt Kahrs is a multisport athlete and celebrity trainer. Some of his long-distance accomplishments include the White River 50 Mile Endurance Run, the 10-mile swim in the Tennessee River, the Delano Park 12 Hour Run, and the Walt Disney World Triathlon. His certifications include Equinox Fitness Tier 3+, Strongfirst Level 1 and 2 Kettlebell, CrossFit Level 2, 500 Hour RYS (Registered Yoga School) Yoga Instructor, and FRC Certified Instructor.

T.E. What was your experience like the first time you did a yin yoga practice?

M.K. I think the first pose I ever did was low dragon. That was intense, because I was coming from a vinyasa flow background. I knew how to get into a pose and be uncomfortable for a short time, but not to sit and simmer in a pose for much longer. That first pose got me. After that, we got into some other postures that felt really good. So, I got both sides, which I love so much about yin yoga. When you come out of it, you're in a whole other mind state, and your body feels really relaxed.

T.E. What would you say to people who are resistant to yin yoga?

M.K. I would say, give it a chance. All that really hard-core training you might be doing, let's say you do circuit training, or you do heavy weight lifting, or you run four or five times a week, you need to balance that out. So that's the biggest thing, is that balance. Yin yoga gives you a chance to hit that reset button and recharge.

T.E. How has yin yoga affected other forms of fitness in your life?

M.K. I'd say the first thing it affected was my other vinyasa yoga classes. I would be in a class, and I'd be like, "Man, I'm more open!" I'm more open in warrior II or warrior I. I can do the binding poses a little better; my spine feels open and my hip flexors feel a little more open. Then it would trickle into some other more hard-core stuff, like if I was running, I felt like my hips weren't locked up as much. Also, in kettlebell training, where you're using your hamstrings a lot, I was able to open up all of that.

T.E. What is your yin yoga practice like these days?

M.K. Sometimes I'll do a straight hour and half yin practice, where I'm picking maybe 5 to 10 poses and sitting in them for 3, 4, or 5 minutes each. Sometimes it'd even be 10 minutes. Then there are those days where I start, and within 20 seconds, I'm already like, "I don't know about this!" [laughter] Again it's a very confronting, challenging type of yoga. When you first do it, it kicks your butt, but you also feel really good at the same time. Usually, after a few times you start to get it, and then after months, you really start to get it. You have to deal with what's mentally, physically, spiritually, and emotionally going on that day.

T.E. What's your favorite yin yoga pose?

M.K. I like seated diamond pose. I get some stretch from it, but I also get a really relaxed feeling. I feel like I can breathe really deep and just chill in that pose for a while.

T.E. What's your least favorite yin yoga pose?

M.K. Least favorite is probably dragon pose. I like it and hate it at the same time. It's the one that if it feels good, I love it. If I don't feel good, and I'm feeling restricted in my hips, in my hamstrings, or my hip flexors, it can be a tough one. I like when I get done with it. I'm like, "Oh man, I made it through that." It's a good challenge.

T.E. Any last "yinspiration" on why yin yoga is important?

M.K. In yin yoga you are checking in with yourself, being quiet, and sitting there. It's kind of like meditation. It balances out that go-go-go type of day that we have with our phones, with our jobs, and with our relationships. You can't get that from any other practice and it's priceless!

CHAPTER 7

DEVELOPING A PERSONAL PRACTICE

"If you commit to nothing, you'll be distracted by everything."
—Tendai Monks

Now that we have explored all the components of yin yoga, the next step is to take action and move into the practice. Understanding the theory is just the beginning, and it is on your yoga mat that the real magic takes place. There is a saying in India that "experience is the greatest guru." In other words, the experience that comes from your yoga practice is the real teacher. Your personal practice will provide you with a lifetime of endless learning, insights, and wisdom.

Your practice is your place to take refuge within the things that are important and meaningful. It is too easy to get swept up within the hecticness of life. In our culture, there are too many things that can pull you away from what is truly important. Your practice is there to reinforce balance internally and externally. The greater your practice, the greater your life will be.

After my knee injury when I got hit by a car, I could have read every book out there on yin yoga, but it wouldn't have healed my body. It was through my personal practice that I engaged my parasympathetic nervous system, regenerated healthy cells, restructured connective tissue, and restored my knee to its natural functioning.

GETTING STARTED

At this point you may have questions. How do I get started? What props do I need? How do I know how often to practice yin yoga? Is it possible to do too much yin? When is the best time to practice? This section answers these questions so you can set up a lifetime of transformative yin practice.

Practice Space

Finding a space for your yin practice can be an exciting experience. Claiming this space as a personal sanctuary will be one of the most powerful actions that you can take for yourself. For some people, it could be an entire room of their home, for others it will be the corner of a room. Wherever it is, make sure it is devoted solely to your yin practice. Remove unnecessary clutter so that it has a spacious quality. Make sure this place is well ventilated to avoid stagnant energy. Keep it clean so that you minimize breathing dust and other particles into the body.

Minimizing noise and distraction in your practice space is also a good idea. Although we don't always have control over our neighbors or even our family members, try to make your space as peaceful as possible. Sometimes turning on a fan or humidifier can produce white noise. If you use a fan, make sure that it's not blowing on you or creating a heavy draft. This can disrupt the air element, which can pull the body and mind away from the yin stillness. Sometimes a Zen-style water fountain can produce the relaxing sound of water to provide a background for quiet relaxation. When it comes to noisy kids and family members, tell them that Travis said to "Quiet down!" Just kidding, but in all seriousness, a brief talk with your significant other, roommates, or kids can be helpful. Explaining to them that this is an important time for you to feed your health and happiness usually will be respected. Because the effects of yin practice greatly decrease tension and stress, family members will beg you to do your practice. From my experience, they won't want to deal with your wrath and fury when you're stressed out. You can also invite your housemates to join in when the time is right. It can be a powerful experience to practice yin with the people that you love.

In our practice space at home, my wife and I have an altar close by. You can put pictures of special people, such as family members or teachers, on your altar. Or you can include pictures that represent the divine. Statues, stones, pure water, symbols, candles, and incense can also be a great addition. Your altar should invoke an energy of benevolence for you.

My meditation teacher, Jack Kornfield, told about an interesting study done in London on the effect that an environment can have on human behavior. A group of researchers chose two streets that were 10 blocks away from each other in a poor, crime-ridden neighborhood in London. They left one street alone and began to transform the other. They picked up trash, painted over the graffiti, and used simple landscaping to enhance the beauty of the street. A year after this project, they went back and looked at the crime statistics for those streets, and the results were astonishing. On the street they had cleaned up, the crime rate dropped 50 percent lower than on the street they had left alone, despite the fact that the streets were only 10 blocks apart.

This study provides insight on how our environment affects our behavior. Most of us know how refreshing it feels when we clear the clutter out of a space and then set it up in an inspiring way. So, take time to set up your practice space and create an environment that feels incredible. The better the vibes, the better your motivation.

Props and Tools

Props, as shown in figure 7.1, are a great addition to your ongoing practice and something that you will be able to use over and over. I highly recommend that you acquire several props to expand your options within the various postures. Having options will ensure that you will be able to find your sweet spot in the pose. Some days you may feel more open and need fewer props. On other days your body may feel tight, and you will use props in every pose.

Yoga Block

I recommend that you get two yoga blocks made of wood or foam. I prefer the lighter foam blocks, especially for a yin practice. The wooden blocks can feel hard and abrasive on the body, which doesn't do much to trigger the relaxation response. If you are new to working with blocks, keep in mind

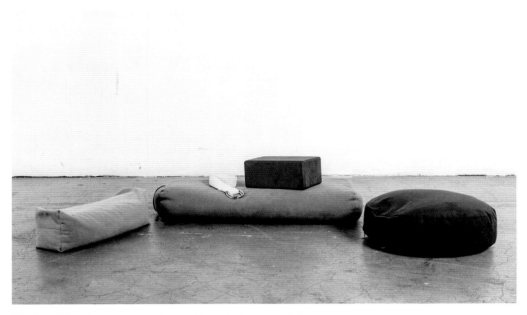

FIGURE 7.1   Yoga props and tools: block, bolsters, and strap.

that each block has three heights. By rotating or turning the block, you can achieve the height that is appropriate for you.

Bolster

A good-quality bolster is a must-have for your practice. Select a bolster that is fairly firm and provides good support. I like the large, rectangular-shaped bolsters as opposed to bolsters that are tube shaped. Although you could get several bolsters, I find that one is enough. You will be able to use the bolster in all sorts of ways to help you find your position. You can also use the bolster as a cushion during meditation and pranayama practices.

Strap

A strap is another useful prop and is used more regularly in a restorative yoga practice. If you find yourself inspired to do a mix of yin and restorative yoga, then I would recommend adding one to your collection. A strap is also helpful during cow face arms pose when the shoulders are tight. Also, if you are stiff in your forward bends, a strap can be helpful. Straps provide leverage to help create a deeper stretch. An example of how this works would be to lasso the strap around the bottom of the foot on the extended leg in half-butterfly pose. Holding the strap with both hands, you can pull yourself into the stretch. As your flexibility improves, you may find that the strap is no longer necessary. In this case, you will reach out and grab the bottom of the foot where the strap used to be positioned.

Blanket

Although you can probably get away without having a blanket, it is definitely worth considering. I prefer the wool blankets commonly found in yoga studios. These can also be used to provide padding. Many people need padding under the back knee in dragon. Sometimes a block or bolster is too thick and the blanket provides an in-between option. You can also place a blanket under the front hip in sleeping swan, and blankets provide comfort in corpse pose. Placing the blanket under the head or even across the belly in a pose like reclining butterfly can take your comfort to a higher level of bliss.

Timer and Music

Using a timer to keep track of time will ensure that you do both sides of the poses evenly. Most smartphones come with a digital stopwatch that you can use as a timer. You can also use a separate stopwatch or the function on your watch if it has one. Because you want to relax as much as possible in your practice, minimize the jarring sounds of a timer going off. I let the stopwatch keep running through my whole practice and do a quick calculation to know when I started and when I need to come out. Over time, your inner clock will become more refined and your intuition will let you know when you're close to finishing. Sometimes, in a difficult pose, it may feel like you have been there for five minutes when in reality you have only been there 50 seconds. This is another reason why tracking your time is important; the clock will hold you accountable for remaining in the position until your time is up. Along those lines, always have a game plan before your practice. Know how long you want to hold the poses. If it is a shorter practice, the holds might be two minutes. If it is a longer practice, then the holds might be five minutes or more.

Playing music in the background of your practice can greatly enhance your enjoyment. Be sure to pick whatever invokes calmness and serenity. Try to have your whole playlist mapped out, so that once you start your practice, you are not in a position of having to act as a DJ. You don't want the music to become a distraction. You want it to enhance the yin qualities of finding stillness and going internal. At other times, practice with no music can provide another kind of powerful exploration. Simple silence can be transformative. Explore and experiment with different techniques to see what feels best. Also, listen to your inner wisdom and, before you practice, see what it is asking for.

If you use your smartphone for music or for a stopwatch, use the airplane mode function. It can be tempting in a long yin pose to get distracted if you can access emails, text messages, and the Internet on your phone. It is inevitable that discomfort or boredom will arise within your practice. Guess what happens the moment your mind becomes bored and restless? It seeks outward stimulation. Where will it get that external stimulation? Your phone! It's too easy. Part of the power of your yin yoga practice is that you are retreating from technology. As we have explored, it is necessary to engage your parasympathetic nervous system, but you can't properly do that if you are looking at your phone or computer or watching TV. Don't make me send the yin police to your house if you violate this rule!

"Almost everything will work again if you unplug it for a few minutes, including you." —Anne Lamott

Frequency and Length of Practice

Determining how often to practice is a personal choice. Everybody is unique. On top of that, each person's bodily requirements change day to day and even moment to moment. Deciding how often to practice is an intuitive decision. The greater your consistency the greater your results, but you can overdo anything, even something as incredible as yin yoga.

Keep in mind that Taoism is all about balance. If you are an athlete who is training hard, then you should strive to balance your hard efforts with a yin yoga practice. This will give the body the important time it needs for full recovery. If you are working hard within your career, then the same advice applies. If you work hard, then also rest hard. Too much yang energy will lead to an imbalance and it never feels good to be sidelined with injury or illness.

For most people, I recommend practicing yin yoga about every other day or three times a week. If you follow this plan, you should experience big shifts within the first month of practice. This could include reduced physical tension, less stress, and an overall sense of wellbeing. Of course, something is better than nothing, so even if you practice once a week, you will see positive changes. During certain times in your life, you may have more time for practice. Take advantage of these opportunities. I've had many students who have been laid off from a job and they see it as a great opportunity to practice more yoga. Practicing yoga keeps them in a clear and positive space until the next job opportunity comes along. When they get the new job, they are happy about their finances, but somewhat sad that they won't have as much time for yoga practice.

When you start a yin yoga practice, I recommend that you cycle through the yin practices offered in this chapter. As they say, variety is the spice of life. It is beneficial to focus on different body areas or themes each time you practice. This will keep your interest high and help you avoid overstressing certain areas. Look at it like a yin style of cross-training.

As you cycle through the sequences several times, you will start to become more accustomed to the various poses and practices. At some point, it will make sense to check in with your body to see what it needs on any given day. If your hips feel tight, then you can do the healthy hips sequence. If

Yin and Restorative Yoga: What's the Difference?

A lot of times when I lead yoga teacher trainings, a common question is asked: What is the difference between yin yoga and restorative yoga? It's a great question because there are many similarities.

Restorative yoga was originated by prolific teacher B.K.S. Iyengar in Pune, India. Iyengar introduced props into the yoga practice as a way to eliminate strain and injury. His method became well known for its attention to alignment. Through the use of props, Iyengar and his teachers were able to modify postures and help students recover from illness and injury. Teacher Judith Hanson Lasater popularized this style of yoga in the United States. The following are the benefits of restorative yoga:

- Decreases the stress hormone cortisol
- Improves sleep, digestion, and immunity
- Releases tense muscles and aching joints
- Teaches conscious control of relaxation
- Increases concentration and focus
- Balances the nervous system
- Activates the relaxation response
- Can act as an introduction to meditation and mindfulness

The aim in restorative yoga is to switch on the relaxation response so that the body's natural ability to rejuvenate and restore itself kicks in. Although this is partially true in yin yoga, the main difference is that in restorative yoga, you never look for an edge or a stretch. As you may remember, looking for the edge is the first step in a yin posture. In restorative yoga, relaxed positions are completely supported by a variety of props to greatly minimize discomfort in the body. In restorative yoga, there is no stretch. In addition to the props suggested earlier in this chapter, restorative yoga often uses sandbags and yoga chairs. In yin yoga, we often hold poses three to five minutes. In restorative yoga, it is common to hold poses for 7 to 10 minutes.

Although the two styles have minor differences, they are much more similar than dissimilar. The intention in both is to slow down, go within, and switch on the parasympathetic nervous system. Of course, any time we use props in our yin yoga practice, we are blending the best of both worlds, combining yin and restorative yoga. Using props will help you to find greater anatomical integrity and therefore avoid bad pain.

you've been traveling in a car or airplane all day and your back is tight, then you can do the flexible-spine sequence. Continue to do the sequences that you tend to avoid. Try to figure out the source of the resistance and be open to exploring the discomfort and challenges. This is often where the biggest breakthroughs come from.

After a year or two of regular practice, you might find yourself beginning to create your own sequences. This is natural and a sign that your relationship to your inner guidance is strong. At this point, go with the flow. If something doesn't work, then you will shift things the next time. Your practice is your laboratory, and exploration and experimentation is a beautiful process. One day you might even find yourself creating a brand-new pose.

When it comes to selecting the length of your practice, 60 minutes should be the target. If you have time to go longer, then by all means indulge yourself with a 90-minute or more practice. I've taught special yin workshops that go two or even three hours. Talk about being blissed out! Those long yin practices will put you into a whole other dimension.

With that said, some days you just don't have time for a long practice. On those days, try for 30 minutes. If 30 minutes is too long, then try 20 minutes. If you are really strapped for time, sneak in a 10-minute yin yoga quickie, choosing four or five postures of about two minutes each. Just make sure that in your shorter practices you do not rush mentally. Whatever your allotted time is, shift into that Taoist state of being and allowing. Sometimes it is more about quality than quantity. Even 10 minutes of quality yin yoga can shift the entire trajectory of your day.

INCORPORATING PRANAYAMA AND MEDITATION INTO YOUR PRACTICE

Bringing pranayama and meditation into your yin practice can take it to a whole new level. In the previous chapter, Pranayama and Meditation, we covered the basics of yoga breathing. In this section, we take it a step further as we incorporate conscious breathing into your regular yin yoga practice.

Let's first explore breathing within the actual yin practice. Different teachers hold different perspectives on how to breathe within a yin posture. Some teachers believe that you should leave the breath alone and let it remain natural and effortless. This is similar to the mindfulness meditation in which you observe the breath without changing its quality. Other teachers support the idea of using a stronger ujjayi type of breath. Deep diaphragmatic breathing can accelerate the process of opening the body. Because the body tissues lengthen during exhalations, emphasizing exhalation will create more space and increase flexibility.

I don't think there is one right way to breathe. It depends on how you feel and what your intention is. If you have had a stressful or emotional day, then it could be helpful to work with big, deep breaths. This will help to release not only tension in the body, but also stress in the mind. The trap for some people, though, is that they push too much during their lives and then they tend to push within their yin poses. This pushing mentality is yang when we want to induce yin. This type of person will benefit from a softer, more effortless breath to practice letting go and letting be.

In my own practice, I adjust the breath to what feels right. In certain positions, I might feel more resistance and therefore will breathe deeper. In an instance like this, I might start with deeper breathing, and then a couple of minutes in, I might shift to a more effortless approach. In some positions that feel sweet and comfortable, I might leave the breath alone the entire time. My advice is to trust yourself. If your inner voice is asking for more breath, then breathe more, and if it is not, then let the breath become natural. Also, anytime you notice your mind wandering in a pose, taking a deeper inhalation can refocus your attention. Keep in mind that working with a gentle ujjayi breath throughout your physical yin practice is considered pranayama.

Traditionally, people start with their physical practice, then move into pranayama practice, and finish with meditation. Each stage prepares them for the next and by the time they get to meditation, they feel completely set up. It can be difficult for people to jump straight into meditation because the mind feels active, busy, and restless. After a good yin practice followed by pranayama, the mind has had sufficient time to adjust.

Although people typically use this sequence, it is OK to explore rearranging the order. Sometimes I start a yin yoga practice with a meditation or pranayama, which can have a powerful effect. Several rounds of a pranayama practice can set the stage for a deep yin yoga practice.

It's been mentioned before, but feel free to explore and see what feels right. I have shared with you many pranayama practices, meditations, poses, and now sequences. You will make great discoveries simply by showing up on your mat and trying different things. Your practice is an inquiry. Ask yourself, "What will happen if I do this today?" Try it and see what happens. It will be amazing, or you will know it doesn't work. Either way, you have gained a new insight and have increased your wisdom. There are no mistakes, only discoveries.

"What you do every day matters more than what you do once in a while." —Gretchen Rubin

INCORPORATING YANG SEQUENCES INTO YOUR PRACTICE

Although this is a yin yoga book, I want to include the following yang sequences as a bonus. Just as yin and yang are complementary qualities, a strong yang sequence can be a great balance for a yin yoga sequence.

Getting the blood flowing and the body warm can be a great way to set up your yin practice. You will encounter less resistance, and your body will naturally be more supple. This can be a great approach when you are practicing first thing in the morning. I rarely roll out of bed, stiff and tight, and say to myself, "Hmmm . . . I feel like doing some yin." Nope, no thank you! I prefer to practice yin yoga after some yang activity or at the end of the day after I've been on the move and need to nourish myself through something long, slow, and deep. Now, that sounds "yinlicious"!

Here you will find five yang sequences: half sun salutation, mountain pose series, sun salutation A, sun salutation B, and the warrior dance flow. Each of these sequences can be done separately or linked with others. The five yang sequences are listed in order of intensity, with half sun salutation being the most gentle and warrior dance flow being the hardest. As mentioned earlier, you can do them separately or you can pick a combination. If you have time, do three or four. If you are short on time, then stick with one or two. Make sure you start with a gentler sequence before progressing to a more difficult one. For example, you would never start with warrior dance flow and then do sun salutation A. Instead, start with sun salutation A and then transition into warrior dance flow. When you are done with your yang sequence, move straight into your preferred yin sequence. These are outlined later in this chapter.

Keep in mind that the yang sequences are optional within your practice. They are not necessary, but they can be a great addition to your practice for the days that you feel inspired to move in an invigorating way. Following are instructions for the five yang sequences.

Half Sun Salutation (Ardha Surya Namaskar)

Half sun salutation is the shortest of the yang sequences. Although it is simple, it effectively loosens both the front and back of the body, especially the hamstrings and low back. It gently promotes circulation of breath and blood. Although it is listed as a yang sequence, it has a sweet yin quality. Treat it as a prayer and meditation in motion. You can flow through this sequence five times or more. This is one of my favorite sequences to do first thing in the morning.

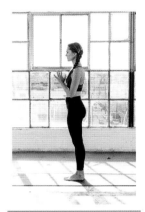 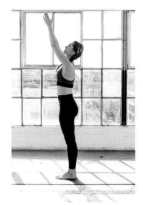 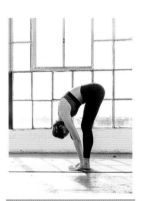 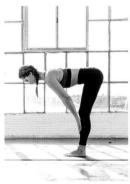

1. Begin in mountain pose with hands in prayer position. Take a few deep breaths in and out through the nose, activating ujjayi breath.

2. Inhale and slowly sweep the arms overhead to upward salute.

3. Exhale and slowly dive down into standing forward bend.

4. Inhale and pull the spine up and out into half forward bend. You can leave the fingers on the floor or bring the hands to the shins.

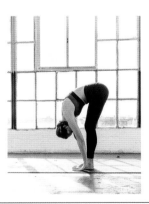 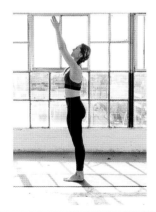 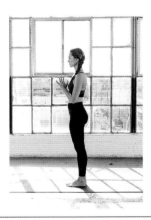

5. Exhale and slowly return to standing forward bend.

6. Inhale and rise to standing and reach the arms overhead.

7. Exhale and return the hands to prayer position in mountain pose.

8. Repeat as often as you like.

Mountain Pose Series (Tadasana)

Mountain pose series has been around for hundreds of years. I first learned it from one of my teachers, Srivatsa Ramaswami, who learned it from his teacher Krishnamacharya. This incredible sequence activates all the major muscle groups in the body through forward bends, backward bends, sideward bends, twists, and more. This series is also said to have a positive effect on each of the seven chakras. Each movement is traditionally repeated three times. This repetition allows the body to open in deeper ways. Every movement starts and finishes in mountain pose. The movements should be slow, steady, and smooth, like a yoga version of tai chi.

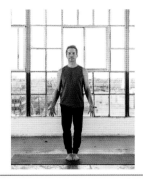

1. Begin in mountain pose by bringing your feet together and relax your arms down by your sides. Close the eyes and find your balance as you feel the soles of the feet evenly rooting into the ground. Begin to take a few steady breaths in and out through the nose, activating ujjayi breath.

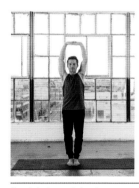
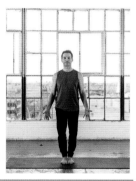
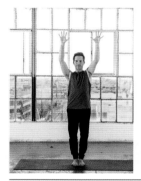
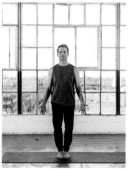

2a. Inhale and slowly sweep the arms overhead, interlacing the fingers and turning the palms facing up.

2b. Exhale and reverse the movement, slowly returning your arms to your sides and into mountain pose. Repeat the movement two more times.

3a. Inhale and bring your arms straight out in front and overhead, with the hands above the shoulders and palms facing forward.

3b. Exhale and reverse the movement, slowly returning your arms to your sides and into mountain pose. Repeat the movement two more times, imagining you're doing the wave at a sporting event.

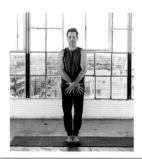
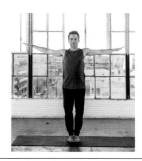
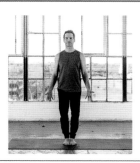

4a. Start with your arms crossed over your abdomen.

4b. Inhale and pull your arms away from each other, with your hands shoulder height. Give the shoulder blades a gentle squeeze at the end of the movement.

4c. Exhale and reverse the movement, this time crossing the opposite arm on top. Then repeat the movement two more times, alternating the cross of the arms each time. At the end of the third cycle, return to mountain pose with arms by your sides.

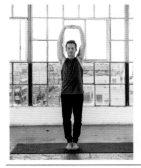
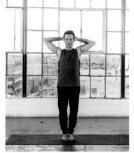
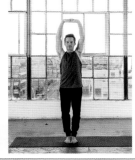
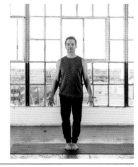

5a. Inhale and slowly sweep the arms overhead, interlacing the fingers and turning the palms facing up.

5b. Exhale and, keeping the fingers interlaced, bring the hands behind the neck, allowing the elbows to flare out.

5c. Inhale and, while keeping the fingers interlaced, straighten the arms back toward the sky.

5d. Exhale and slowly return the arms to mountain pose. Repeat the movement two more times.

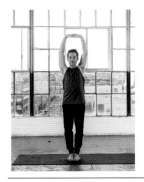
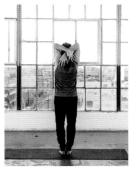
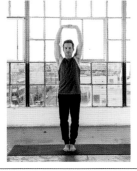
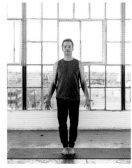

6a. Inhale and slowly sweep the arms overhead, interlacing the fingers and turning the palms facing up.

6b. Exhale and bring opposite hands to opposite shoulder blades, with the elbows facing upward.

6c. Inhale, interlace the fingers, and stretch the arms toward the sky.

6d. Exhale and slowly return the arms down to mountain pose. Repeat the movement two more times, alternating the cross of the arms each time.

(continued)

Mountain Pose Series (Tadasana)

(continued)

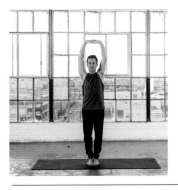

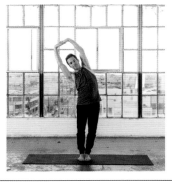

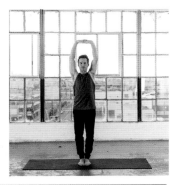

7a. Inhale and slowly sweep the arms overhead, interlacing the fingers and turning the palms facing up.

7b. Exhale and side-bend to the right.

7c. Inhale and return to center.

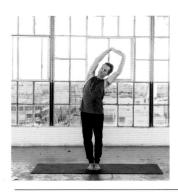

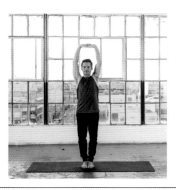

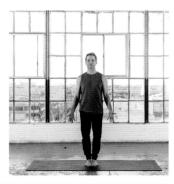

7d. Exhale and side-bend to the left.

7e. Inhale and return to center.

7f. Exhale and slowly return the arms to mountain pose. Repeat two more times. On the third round, hold the side-bend stretch for three or four breaths, emphasizing the stretch.

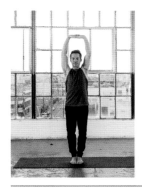 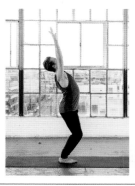 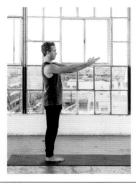 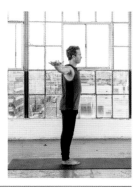

8a. Inhale and slowly sweep the arms overhead, interlacing the fingers and turning the palms facing up.

8b. Exhale and separate the hands shoulder-width apart while bending the knees and arching back.

8c. On the same exhale, straighten the legs and sweep the arms around to the front with the palms facing up.

8d. Inhale and spread the arms out to the side.

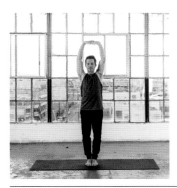 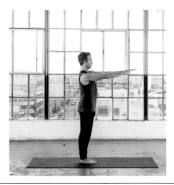 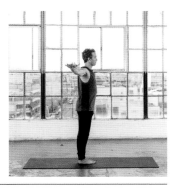

8e. Sweep the arms overhead, interlacing the fingers and turning the palms facing up.

8f. Exhale and lower the arms to shoulder height with the palms facing down.

8g. Spread the arms out to the side.

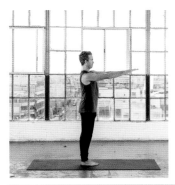 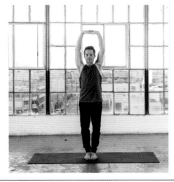 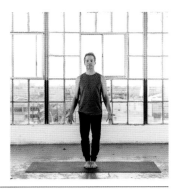

8h. Inhale and bring the arms back out in front.

8i. Reach the arms overhead, interlace the fingers, and turn the palms facing up.

8j. Exhale and slowly return the arms to your sides into mountain pose. Repeat two more times.

(continued)

Mountain Pose Series (Tadasana)

(continued)

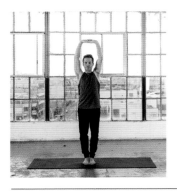 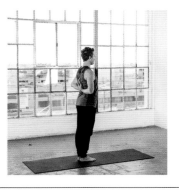 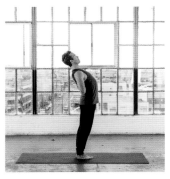

9a. Inhale and slowly sweep the arms overhead, interlacing the fingers and turning the palms facing up.

9b. Exhale and bring the hands around the back to reverse prayer, with the palms touching and the fingers facing upward.

9c. If you need to modify, press your fists together. Inhale, lean back, and gently look up.

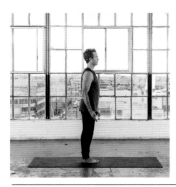 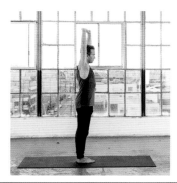 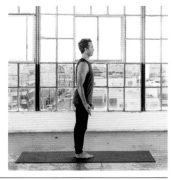

9d. Exhale, return to face forward, and release the arms to your sides.

9e. Inhale and slowly sweep the arms overhead, interlacing the fingers and turning the palms facing up.

9f. Exhale and slowly return the arms to your sides into mountain pose. Repeat two more times. On the third round, hold the reverse prayer backbend and take three or four breaths.

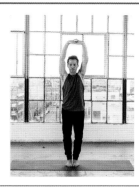 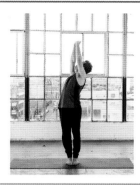 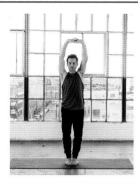

10a. Inhale and slowly sweep the arms overhead, interlacing the fingers and turning the palms facing up.

10b. Exhale and twist to the right, gently arching back and looking up.

10c. Inhale and rotate to face the front.

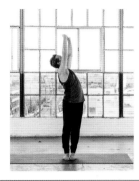 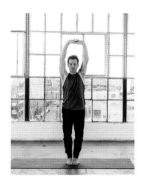 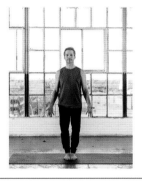

10d. Exhale and twist to the left, gently arching back and looking up.

10e. Inhale and rotate to face the front.

10f. Exhale and slowly return the arms to your sides into mountain pose. Repeat two more times. During the third round, hold the twist and arch back while taking three or four breaths.

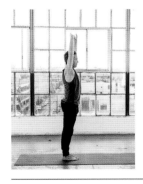 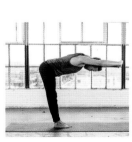 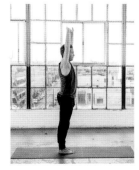 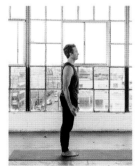

11a. Inhale and slowly sweep the arms overhead, interlacing the fingers and turning the palms facing up.

11b. Exhale and, keeping the fingers interlaced, fold halfway over. Feel the hips draw back as the palms press forward.

11c. Inhale and bring the arms back overhead.

11d. Exhale and slowly return the arms to mountain pose. Repeat two more times. On the third round, hold the half forward bend and take three or four breaths.

(continued)

Mountain Pose Series (Tadasana)

(continued)

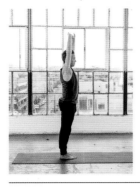 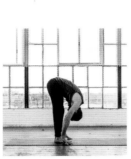 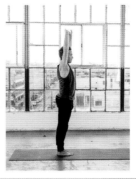 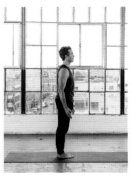

12a. Inhale and slowly sweep the arms overhead, interlacing the fingers and turning the palms facing up.

12b. Exhale, separate the hands shoulder-width apart, and fold all the way over into a forward bend.

12c. Inhale and, while staying low, interlace the fingers and then rise all the way up with the arms overhead.

12d. Exhale and slowly return the arms to mountain pose. Repeat two more times. During the third round, hold the forward bend and take three or four breaths.

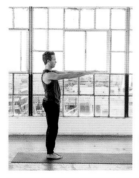 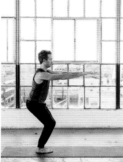 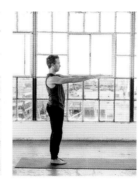 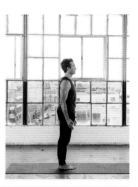

13a. Inhale and lift the arms straight out in front, with the hands shoulder height and facing down.

13b. Exhale, bend the knees, and lower into a half squat.

13c. Inhale, straighten the legs, and return to standing.

13d. Exhale and return the arms to the sides into mountain pose. Repeat two more times. On the third round, hold the half squat and take three or four breaths.

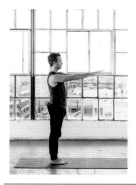 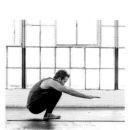 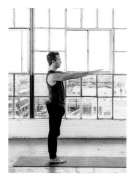 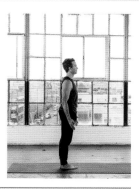

14a. Inhale and lift the arms straight out in front, with the hands shoulder height and facing down.

14b. Exhale, bend the knees, and lower into a full squat.

14c. Inhale, straighten the legs, and return to standing.

14d. Exhale and slowly return the arms to the sides into mountain pose. Repeat two more times. On the third round, hold the full squat and take three or four breaths.

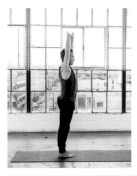 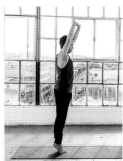 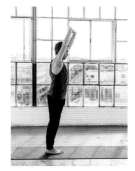 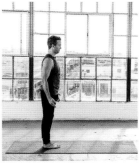

15a. Inhale and slowly sweep the arms overhead, interlacing the fingers and turning the palms facing up.

15b. Exhale, lift the heels, and balance on the tips of the toes.

15c. Inhale and return the heels to the floor.

15d. Exhale and slowly return the arms to the sides in mountain pose. Repeat two more times. During the third round, hold the toe balance and take three or four breaths.

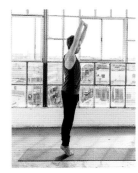 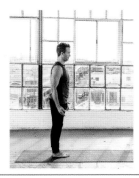

16a. Inhale and slowly sweep the arms overhead, interlacing the fingers and at the same time balancing on the tips of the toes.

16b. Exhale and slowly lower both the arms and heels. Repeat two more times. On the third round, hold the toe balance and take three or four breaths.

Sun Salutations (Surya Namaskar)

Both of the following sun salutations are a great way to warm up the body and produce a yang effect. More vigorous than the mountain pose (tadasana) series, these sequences are often experienced in a vinyasa or power yoga practice. The poses will strengthen and lengthen major muscle groups. As you move through the poses, the heart rate will quicken, increasing blood circulation through the body and providing a cardio effect. To prevent injuries, it is advisable to learn the proper alignment for the poses from a qualified instructor. Take your time for the first round of each sun

SUN SALUTATION A

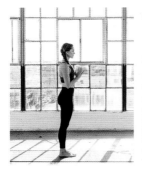 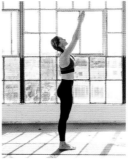 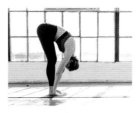 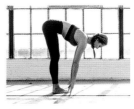

1. Begin in mountain pose with hands in prayer position. Take a few deep breaths in and out through the nose, activating ujjayi breath.

2. Inhale and sweep the arms overhead to upward salute.

3. Exhale and dive into standing forward bend.

4. Inhale and pull the spine up and out into half forward bend. You can leave the fingers on the floor or bring the hands to the shins.

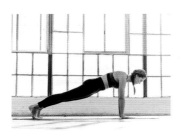 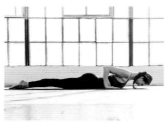 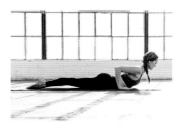

5a. Exhale and step back into a push-up position for plank.

5b. On the same exhalation, lower slowly to the ground using the upper-body muscles.

6. Inhale and lift the chest and slide the shoulders back into cobra.

salutation. In the first round, the setup round, take a few breaths in each pose. Here you can focus on proper alignment. After you have moved through the setup round, you can flow through it for another two to four cycles. During the flow cycles, coordinate one breath with one movement. In India, these sequences are used as an expression of giving gratitude and honoring the sun for its light and energy. While flowing through the movements, explore bringing a devotional quality so that it becomes a moving prayer.

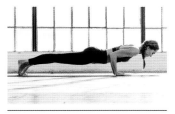

7. Exhale and press into a push-up and come in to downward dog (p. 162).

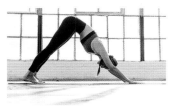

8. Inhale and press the hips back in downward dog.

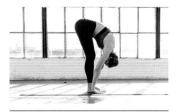

9. Exhale and step both feet forward into standing forward bend.

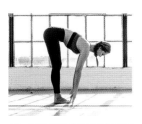

10. Inhale and pull the spine up and out into half forward bend.

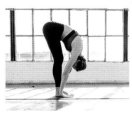

11. Exhale and release the torso into standing forward bend.

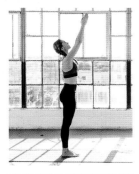

12. Inhale and rise to standing and sweep the arms overhead into upward salute.

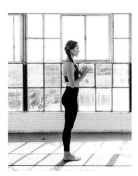

13. Exhale and return to mountain pose, with the hands in prayer position. Repeat steps 1 through 13 two to four more times, linking the breath with the movement.

(continued)

Sun Salutations (Surya Namaskar)

(continued)

SUN SALUTATION B

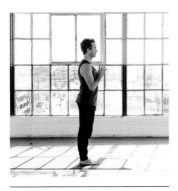

1. Begin in mountain pose, with hands in prayer position. Take a few deep breaths in and out through the nose, activating ujjayi breath.

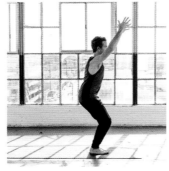

2. Inhale and bend the knees, squat back, and lift the arms overhead into chair.

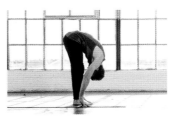

3. Exhale and dive into standing forward bend.

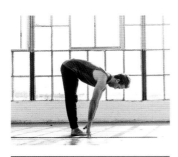

4. Inhale and pull the spine up and out into half forward bend. Leave the fingers on the floor or bring the hands to the shins.

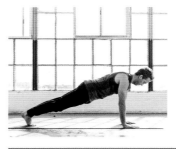

5a. Exhale and step back into a push-up position for plank.

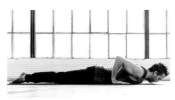

5b. On the same exhalation, lower slowly to the ground using the upper-body muscles.

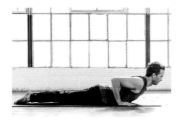

6. Inhale and lift the chest up and slide the shoulders back into cobra.

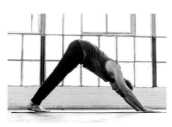

7. Exhale, push into a push-up, and draw the hips back into downward dog.

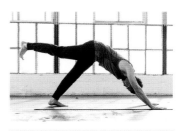

8. Inhale and lift the right leg parallel to the floor into three-legged downward dog.

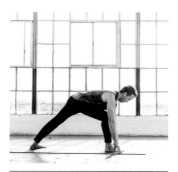

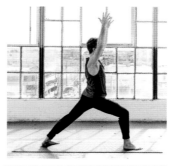

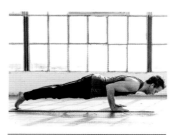

9. Exhale and step the right foot forward between the hands and turn the back foot, keeping it flat to the mat.

10. Inhale and rise to standing with the arms reaching up into warrior I.

11. Exhale and lower the hands to the floor, step the right foot back, and lower with control to the floor.

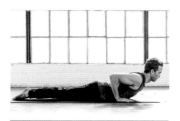

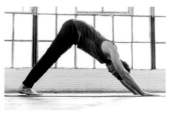

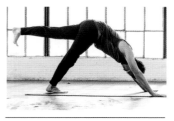

12. Inhale and lift the chest and slide the shoulders back into cobra.

13. Exhale, press into a push-up, and draw the hips back into downward dog.

14. Inhale and lift the left leg parallel to the floor into three-legged downward dog.

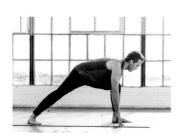

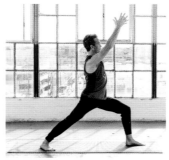

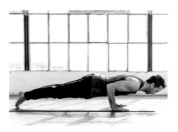

15. Exhale and step the left foot forward between the hands and turn the back foot, keeping it flat to the mat.

16. Inhale and rise to standing, with the arms reaching up into warrior I.

17. Exhale and lower the hands to the floor, step the left foot back, and lower with control to the floor.

(continued)

235

Sun Salutations (Surya Namaskar)

(continued)

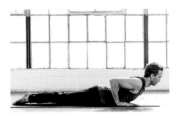

18. Inhale and lift the chest and slide the shoulders back into cobra.

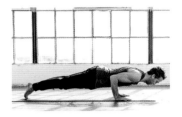

19. Exhale, and come into downward dog (page 162) and press into a push-up.

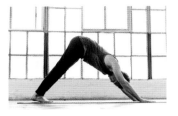

20. Inhale and press the hips back in downward dog.

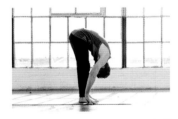

21. Exhale and step both feet forward into standing forward bend.

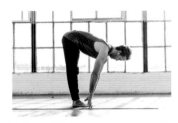

22. Inhale and pull the spine up and out into half forward bend.

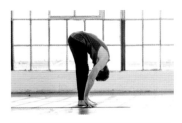

23. Exhale and release the torso into standing forward bend.

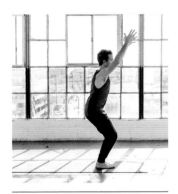

24. Inhale and bend the knees, squat back, and lift the arms into chair.

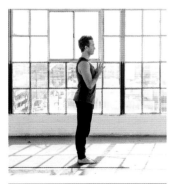

25. Exhale and stand up, returning to mountain pose with the hands in prayer position. Repeat steps 1 through 25 two to four more times.

Warrior Dance Flow

The warrior dance flow is a fun and invigorating continuation of sun salutations A and B. For those days when you feel like you have extra stress to release, you can move directly into this sequence after sun salutations A and B. Just as in the previous two sequences, allow the first round to be your setup cycle where you take your time to focus on the alignment. Next, focus on rhythm and finding your flow. The intention of this sequence is to tap into the strength and power of the warrior. Enjoy!

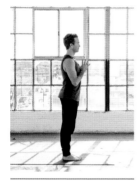
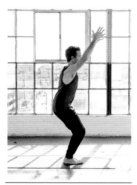
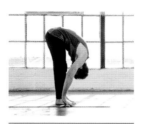
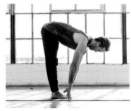

1. Picking up at the end of sun salutation B, start in mountain pose with hands at prayer.

2. Inhale, bend the knees to squat back, and lift the arms into chair.

3. Exhale and dive into standing forward bend.

4. Inhale and pull the spine up and out into half forward bend.

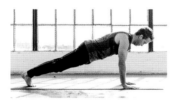
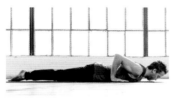
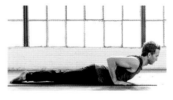

5a. Exhale and step back into a push-up position for plank.

5b. On the same exhalation, lower slowly to the ground using the upper-body muscles.

6. Inhale and lift the chest and slide the shoulders back into cobra.

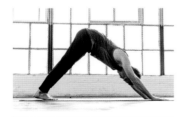
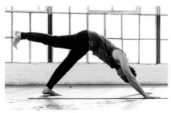
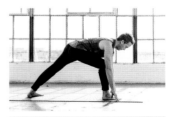

7. Exhale, press into a push-up, and draw the hips back into downward dog.

8. Inhale and lift the right leg parallel to the floor into three-legged downward dog.

9. Exhale and step the right foot forward between the hands and turn the back foot, keeping it flat to the mat.

(continued)

Warrior Dance Flow

(continued)

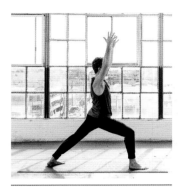

10. Inhale and rise to standing, with the arms reaching up into warrior I.

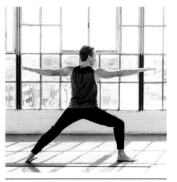

11. Exhale and open the chest to the left and spread the arms into warrior II.

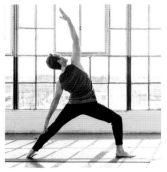

12. Inhale and rotate the front palm up, lean back, and place the left hand on the back leg, moving into reverse warrior.

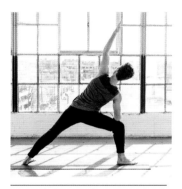

13. Exhale and move back through warrior II, rest the right forearm on top on the front thigh, and extend the top arm forward into modified extended side angle.

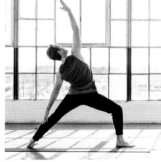

14. Inhale and return to reverse warrior.

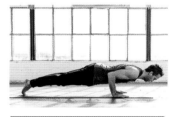

15. Exhale and windmill the hands to the floor, step the right foot back, and lower with control to the floor.

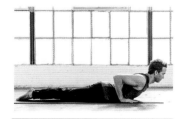

16. Inhale and lift the chest and slide the shoulders back into cobra.

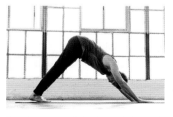

17. Exhale, press into a push-up, and draw the hips back into downward dog.

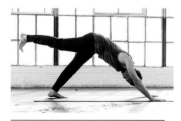

18. Inhale and lift the left leg parallel to the floor into three-legged downward dog.

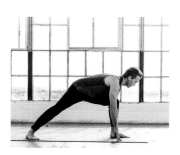

19. Exhale and step the left foot forward between the hands and turn the back foot, keeping it flat to the mat.

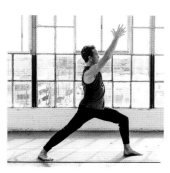

20. Inhale and rise to standing, with the arms reaching up into warrior I.

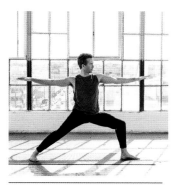

21. Exhale and open the chest to the right and spread the arms into warrior II.

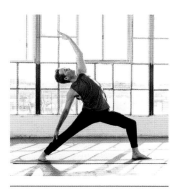

22. Inhale and rotate the front palm up, lean back, and place the right hand on the back leg, moving into reverse warrior.

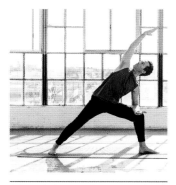

23. Exhale and move back through warrior II, rest the left forearm on top on the front thigh, and extend the top arm forward into modified extended side angle.

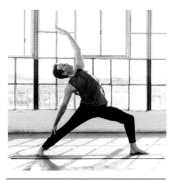

24. Inhale and return to reverse warrior.

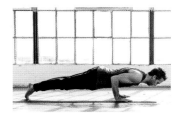

25. Exhale and windmill the hands to the floor, step the left foot back, and lower with control to the floor.

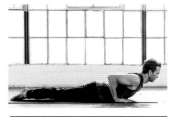

26. Inhale and lift the chest and slide the shoulders back into cobra.

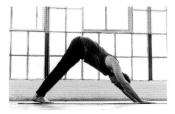

27. Exhale, press into a push-up, and draw the hips back into downward dog. Repeat steps 7 through 27 two to four more times.

JOURNEYING INTO YOUR YIN YOGA PRACTICE

This is where it all comes together! Are you excited? I'm assuming that if you made it this far in the book that you are. I know that I am. I can't wait for you to put your yin pedal to the yin metal!

In this section, I share 10 powerful and thematic practices. This is where we take all the poses from chapter 5 and put them to good use. My hope is that this section provides you tremendous value and variety so that you will experience the magnificent practice of yin. Each sequence is specially crafted to explore different areas in the body. You can hold the yin poses in these sequences for 90 seconds to 5 minutes, depending on your needs. Typically, the longer you practice, the closer to five minutes you should hold. Keep in mind that the counterstretches, which are more yang in nature, are usually held for about five breaths. Also, poses like legs up the wall, supported bridge, and corpse pose can easily be held for more than five minutes.

I recommend that you start with sequence 1 and take your time working up to sequence 10. Enjoy the journey, there is no rush. It is yin yoga after all. Like Lao Tzu says, "Nature does not hurry, yet everything is accomplished." After you have completed the entire rotation, you can go back and pick sequences a la carte, depending on what your needs are on any given day. Once your practice space is set up, grab this book, take it to your mat, and let's go yin deep!

"It is not the daily increase but the daily decrease. Hack away the inessentials." —Bruce Lee

Yin Sequence 1: Short and Sweet

This basic sequence is great for beginners or when time is short. Yin short and sweet provides simple but sweet stretches for the spine, hips, and inner thighs.

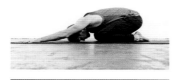

1. Child's pose (page 102)

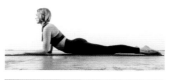

2. Sphinx pose (page 127)

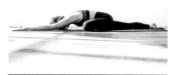

3. Sleeping swan, each side (page 123)

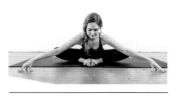

4. Butterfly pose (page 93)

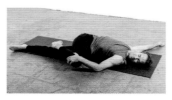

5. Reclining twist, each side (page 148)

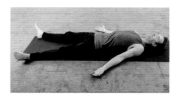

6. Corpse pose (page 152)

Yin Sequence 2: Ultimate

This sequence is a personal favorite that evenly stretches the hips and the spine, and maintains healthy knees.

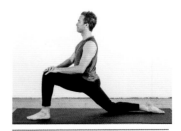

1. Child's pose (page 102)

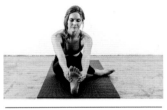

2. Downward dog (page 162)

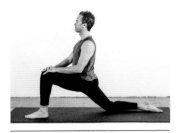

3. Dragon pose, first side (page 128)

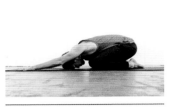

4. Sleeping swan, first side (page 123)

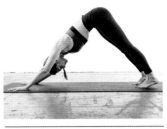

5. Half shoelace, first side (page 125) or half-butterfly pose, first side (page 94)

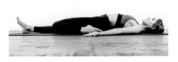

6. Reclining half hero, first side (page 117)

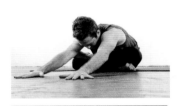

7. Fire log pose, first side (page 126)

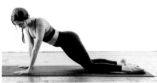

8. Hip circles, both directions (page 168)

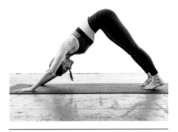

9. Downward dog (page 162)

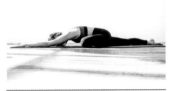

10. Dragon pose, second side (page 128)

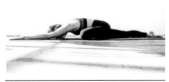

11. Sleeping swan, second side (page 123)

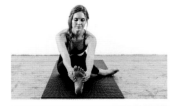

12. Half shoelace, second side (page 125) or half-butterfly pose, second side (page 94)

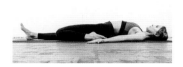

13. Reclining half hero, second side (page 117)

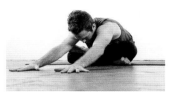

14. Fire log pose, second side (page 128)

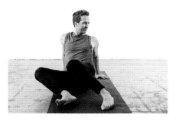

15. Windshield wipers (page 170)

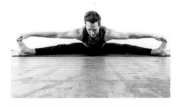

16. Dragonfly pose (page 96)

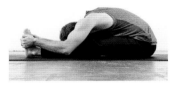

17. Caterpillar pose (page 92)

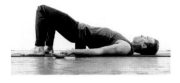

18. Supported bridge (page 143)

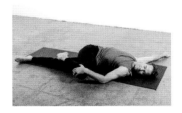

19. Reclining twist, each side (page 148)

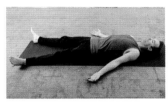

20. Corpse pose (page 152)

Yin Sequence 3: Flexible Spine

This sequence focuses on the health and well-being of the spine. It includes forward bends, backward bends, sideways bends, twists, and an inversion. This practice is especially beneficial for your brain.

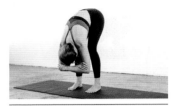

1. Dangling standing forward bend (page 108)

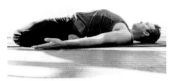

2. Saddle pose (page 115)

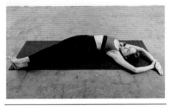

3. Banana pose, each side (page 144)

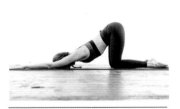

4. Melting heart (page 103)

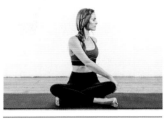

5. Easy seated twist, each side (page 120)

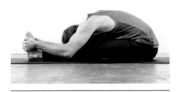

6. Caterpillar pose (page 92)

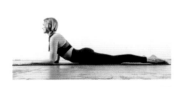

7. Sphinx pose (page 127) or seal pose (page 134)

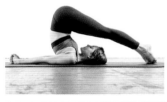

8. Snail pose (page 146)

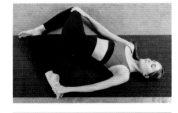

9. Cat pulling its tail pose, each side (page 150)

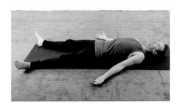

10. Corpse pose (page 152)

Yin Sequence 4: Healthy Hips

This sequence stretches the hips in various positions to ensure that the largest joint in your body is healthy and open.

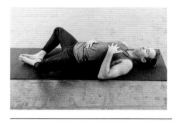

1. Reclining butterfly (page 136) or reclining tepee (page 137)

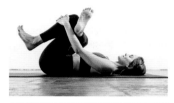

2. Reclining pigeon, first side (page 140)

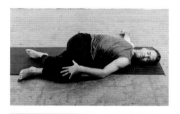

3. Reclining wrap-leg twist, first side (page 149)

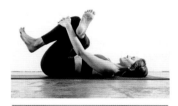

4. Reclining pigeon, second side (page 140)

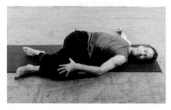

5. Reclining wrap-leg twist, second side (page 149)

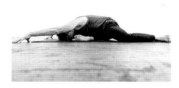

6. Deer pose, first side (page 122)

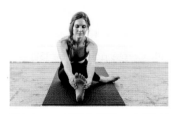

7. Half shoelace, first side (page 125) or half-butterfly pose, first side (page 94)

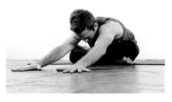

8. Fire log pose, first side (page 126) or easy seated pose, first side (page 118)

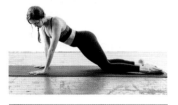

9. Hip circles, each direction (page 168)

(continued)

Yin Sequence 4: Healthy Hips

(continued)

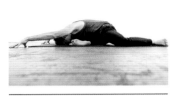

10. Deer pose, second side (page 122)

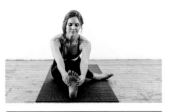

11. Half shoelace, second side (page 125) or half-butterfly pose, second side (page 94)

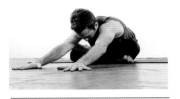

12. Fire log pose, second side (page 126) or easy seated pose, second side (page 118)

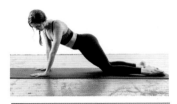

13. Hip circles, each direction (page 168)

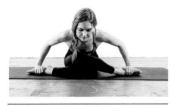

14. Shoelace pose, each side (page 124)

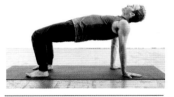

15. Upward table, pulse 5 times (page 163)

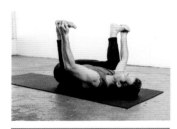

16. Stirrup pose (page 142)

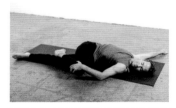

17. Reclining twist, each side (page 148)

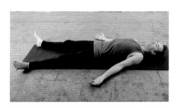

18. Corpse pose (page 152)

Yin Sequence 5: Sleep Well

This sequence starts with gentle yoga to sweetly open the body. It finishes with yin postures to prepare the body for a night's deep sleep.

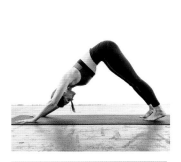

1. Resting belly pose (page 132)

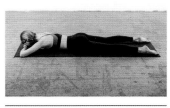
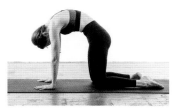

2. Cat and cow for 10 cycles (page 164)

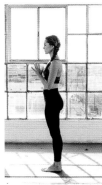

3. Downward dog (page 162)

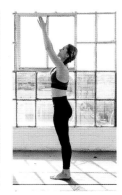
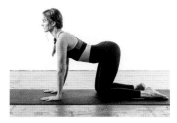
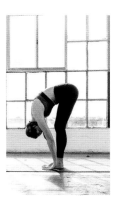

4. Half sun salutation for 5 cycles (page 223)

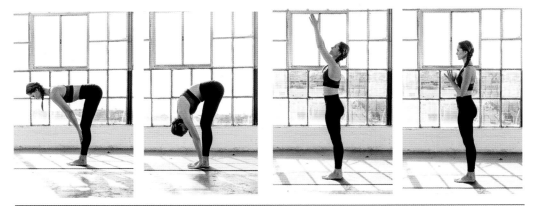

4. Half sun salutation for 5 cycles (page 223)

(continued)

Yin Sequence 5: Sleep Well

(continued)

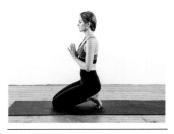

5. Toe squat pose (page 112)

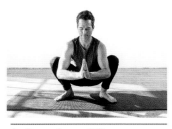

6. Squat (page 110)

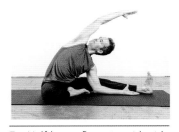

7. Half-butterfly pose with side stretch, first side (pages 94-95)

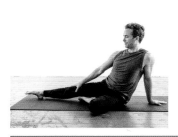

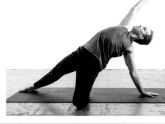

8. Half-butterfly backbend for 5 cycles, first side (page 166)

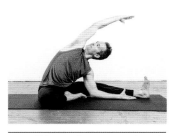

9. Half-butterfly pose with side stretch, second side (pages 94-95)

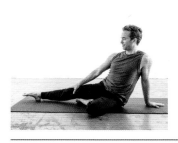

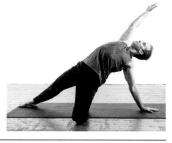

10. Half-butterfly backbend for 5 cycles, second side (page 166)

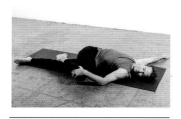

11. Reclining twist, each side (page 148)

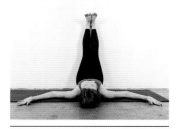

12. Legs up the wall (page 151)

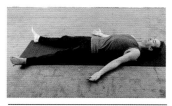

13. Corpse pose (page 152)

Yin Sequence 6: Splits

This sequence prepares the body for variations of the splits.

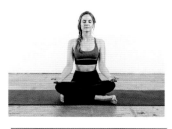

1. Easy seated pose (sit on a block if needed) (page 118)

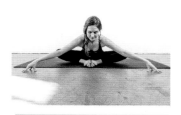

2. Butterfly pose (page 93)

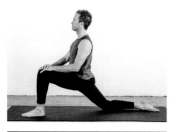

3. Dragon pose (shown here), low dragon pose, or angled low dragon pose, each side (page 129)

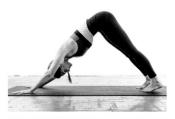

4. Downward dog (page 162)

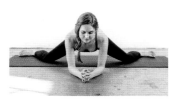

5. Frog pose (page 98)

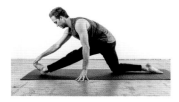

6. Half splits (shown here) or full splits, each side (page 130)

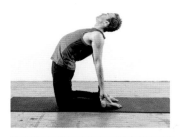

7. Camel pose (page 104)

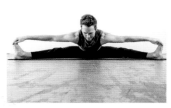

8. Dragonfly pose (page 96)

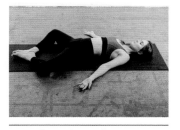

9. Reclining butterfly (page 136)

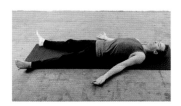

10. Corpse pose (page 152)

Yin Sequence 7: For Athletes

This series is designed for athletes to promote rest and recovery throughout the body.

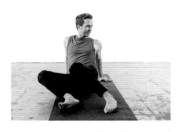

1. Reclining tree, each side (page 138)

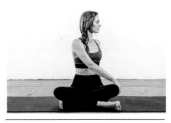

2. Easy seated twist, each side (page 120)

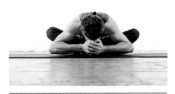

3. Seated diamond pose (page 121)

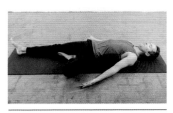

4. Windshield wipers (page 170)

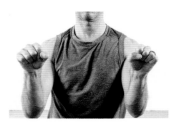

5. Wrist stretch sequence (page 158)

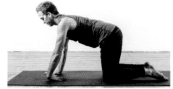

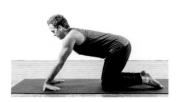

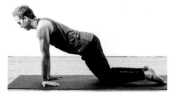

5. Wrist stretch sequence (page 158)

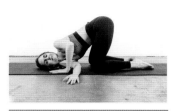

6. Thread-the-needle shoulder stretch, each side (page 106)

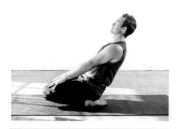

7. Ankle stretch (page 114)

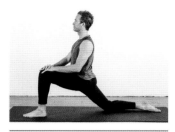

8. Dragon pose (shown here) or angled low dragon pose, each side (page 129)

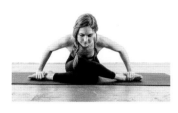

9. Shoelace pose, each side (page 124)

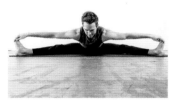

10. Dragonfly pose (page 96)

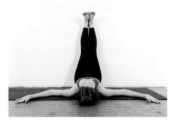

11. Legs up the wall (page 151)

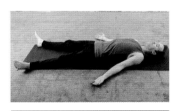

12. Corpse pose (page 152)

Yin Sequence 8: Yin and Tonic

This sequence is guaranteed to take the edge off after a long, stressful day. Allow your body to decrease stressors and increase feel-good chemicals the natural way.

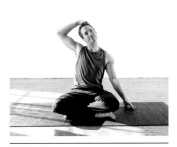

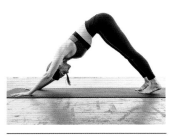

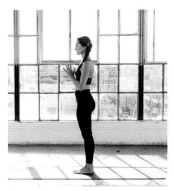

1. Easy seated pose with lateral neck stretch, each side (page 154)

2. Downward dog (page 162)

3. Half sun salutation for 5 cycles (page 223)

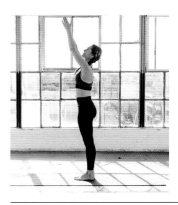

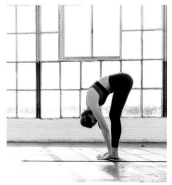

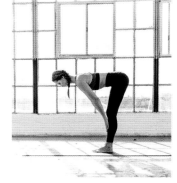

3. Half sun salutation for 5 cycles (page 223)

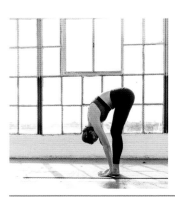

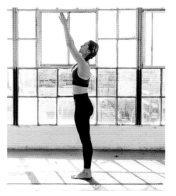

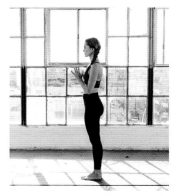

3. Half sun salutation for 5 cycles (page 223)

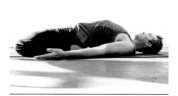

4. Saddle pose (page 115) or hero pose (page 116)

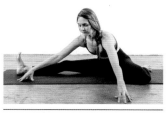

5. Half-frog pose, each side (page 100)

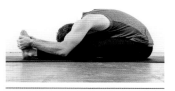

6. Caterpillar pose (page 92)

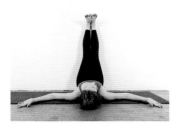

7. Reclining pigeon, each side (page 140)

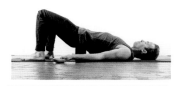

8. Supported bridge (page 143)

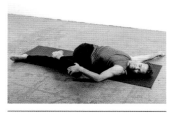

9. Reclining twist, each side (page 148)

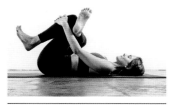

10. Legs up the wall (page 151)

Yin Yoga Sequence 9: Upper Body

Most of time, the hips and the spine get the majority of the love in yin yoga. This sequence spreads the yin medicine into the upper body, including the neck, chest, shoulders, and wrists.

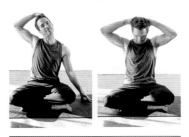

1. Easy seated pose with lateral and forward neck stretches (pages 154 and 153)

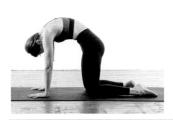

2. Cat and cow for 10 cycles (page 164)

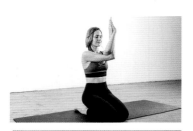

3. Hero pose supported on a block (pages 116 and 184) with eagle arms, each side (page 160)

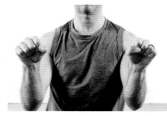

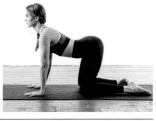

4. Wrist stretch sequence (page 158)

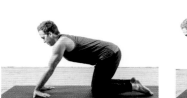

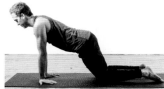

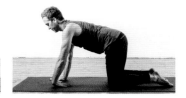

4. Wrist stretch sequence (page 158)

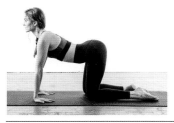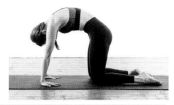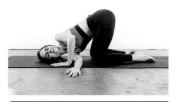

5. Cat and cow with reversed hands for 10 cycles (page 164)

6. Thread-the-needle shoulder stretch, each side (page 106)

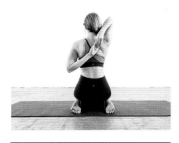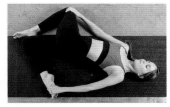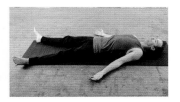

7. Hero pose supported on a block (pages 116 and 184) with cow face arms, each side (page 156)

8. Cat pulling its tail pose, each side (page 150)

9. Corpse pose (page 152)

Yin Sequence 10: Prenatal

This series was designed by pre- and postnatal expert instructor Desi Bartlett. This series prepares mothers-to-be for childbirth by opening the hips, releasing tension in the back, and triggering the relaxation response. Even if you are not pregnant, it is a great sequence, so give it a go.

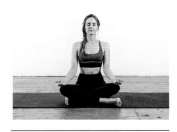

1. Easy seated pose (page 118)

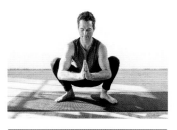

2. Squat (page 110)

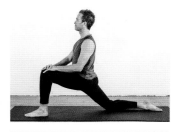

3. Dragon pose, each side (page 128)

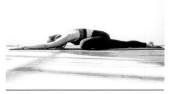

4. Sleeping swan, each side (page 123)

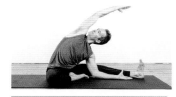

5. Half-butterfly pose with side stretch, each side (pages 94-95)

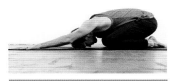

6. Child's pose with wide knees and bolster under forehead (page 102)

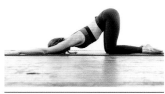

7. Melting heart with forearms on top of two blocks and forehead relaxed on the bolster between the arms (page 103)

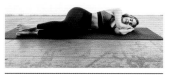

8. Corpse pose on left side with a bolster or blanket between the knees (page 152).

Our journey together is almost complete. Now that you have multiple sequences, I encourage you to try them out. I hope you enjoy them and receive many benefits from your yin practice. Before we wrap things up, join me in the next chapter for inspiration and final thoughts.

Dana Byerlee

Dana is a writer and meditation and yoga teacher based in Los Angeles. As a cancer survivor, Dana has a passion for studying the mind–body–spirit connection. Her mission is to help people embrace their lives fully and with an open heart.

T.E. Can you share a little of your backstory?

D.B. I used to live in New York, working in the corporate world. Sometimes it would be 17-hour days, and then going out drinking, not eating properly, and not sleeping well. Back then I thought the only way to be successful and to achieve things was to be in burnout mode all the time. After moving to San Francisco, I noticed a lump, and then it was diagnosed as a cancerous mass. At the time, all I did was have a lumpectomy and tried to change my diet and lifestyle. I embraced a much more alkaline diet. I moved to LA, and I went to a yoga class of yours. You were talking about a yoga teacher training and something told me, "Oh, that'd be good. I need this for my health and for the long term." After that fall training, I went back to the doctor and the lump had come back. This time I had to take a different action. Along with the Western approach of chemotherapy and surgery, now I also had the tools from yoga and meditation. This helped me to be with uncomfortable physical things and uncomfortable emotions like fear.

T.E. When did you do yin yoga the first time and what was it like?

D.B. It was in teacher training. It was really confronting and intense. I'm not intrinsically the most flexible, so there was that point of not wanting to hold things for that long and wanting to really run away. Seeing the difference of holding something 30 seconds and up to four or five minutes was so confronting. Even though it was a really difficult practice, there were a couple of moments where I was able to use my breath as that ladder to extend and then deepen. When I actually shut off the mental and physical resistance, I noticed how the body began to relax into the pose.

T.E. How did the insights from your practice support you during your treatment phase?

D.B. I explored what would happen if I just stood out of the way as much as possible. Something I learned from yin and the Tao is that nature's power is its patience. So, could I have the patience to let the treatment run its course? That was huge. During these times, especially in between treatments, yin was all I could do. I feel like those practices kept my body in a better state, kept me more supple. I think yin yoga kept the chi flowing in a more balanced way.

T.E. What's your favorite yin yoga pose?

D.B. Shoelace.

T.E. What is your least favorite yin yoga pose?

D.B. I would say dragonfly pose.

T.E. What is the biggest takeaway from your transition from the high-achieving corporate Dana from the past and who you are now?

D.B. I think the wisdom that not all movement and progress comes just from the things that we can see and control. There's a natural wisdom at work. Our body's innate healing system is at work. Also, letting myself have a bit more flow to life instead of pushing and forcing. It's allowing myself to be led different places. I used to feel that might sound passive or not being responsible. But it is true there's a lot more flow and synchronicity. I don't know what you call it, maybe natural magic. I've definitely lightened my foot off the gas pedal!

CHAPTER 8
INSPIRATION AND FINAL THOUGHTS

"I wish I could show you, when you are lonely or in darkness, the astonishing light of your own being."

—Hafiz

We are coming to the end of our journey together. When you reflect on all that we've explored, it has been a full immersion into the wonderful world of yin yoga. As you can now clearly see, the subject of yin yoga is immensely deep. Thousands of years ago, it was the first physical yoga. It provided the support for yogis on the path of liberation and awakening. This was a liberation from unnecessary misery and suffering. This was an awakening to the Tao that is infinite and indestructible. Through the various practices of yoga and Taoism, the inner forces of chi were summoned, harnessed, and channeled for the practitioner to reach the pinnacle of human experience. Whether you are passionate about the mystical or the scientific or perhaps both, it's undeniable that the practice of yin yoga is magnificent. And this is because human life is sacred and magnificent. Yin yoga and the philosophy of Taoism are merely a way of allowing this magnificence to flourish.

Human life is a wild ride with all the gain and loss, health and sickness, sweetness and challenge that we all face. Life isn't always easy. Sometimes it is, and we find ourselves in a great flow where everything seems to click along the way we would like it to. Other times, it's a different story. We struggle to put our best foot forward as we face challenges on all fronts: our relationships, health, career, and finances. As the Tao teaches, everything is impermanent.

While writing this book, I faced an intense lesson on impermanence. Halfway through the writing process on a Sunday morning, I popped open my laptop to begin a writing session. I clicked to open the document. After several seconds had passed and the file had loaded, I was aghast that almost 100 pages were missing. Basically, everything that I had written during an entire month was gone in an instant. Everything that I had sacrificed to write during that month flooded through my mind. I thought about all the hours that I had stepped away from my family, my yoga practice, and my downtime to work on the book.

Despite autosave and visiting the Apple Store and the Microsoft Store, no expert could retrieve the lost pages. They were gone, and I was distraught. I was so upset that I was going to walk away from this book altogether. Luckily, my wife talked some sense into me and steered me back onto the path after I was dangerously close to jumping off the cliff. As famed basketball coach John Wooden said, "Show me your friends, and I'll show you your future" (Wooden, 2016). I was fortunate to have a loving wife and a compassionate editor to ensure that my future involved completing this book. Had it not been for them, you and I might not have gotten to share this journey together.

So, this is the way life is and we can all relate to what it feels like to lose something. Of course, losing a loved one is way more shattering than losing a physical object or 100 pages of a book. But this is the ticket we purchased for the ride of human incarnation. Our yin yoga practice brings us back to the center of who we are. It brings us back to wisdom, steadiness, and knowingness.

Often as we move through the inevitable challenges of life, we can feel isolated and alone. Surrounding ourselves with uplifting people serves as a constant reminder that we have support. Sometimes we get lost within the darkness of despair, especially when we move through a personal tragedy. Our friends and loved ones can help bring us back into the light. Sometimes all it takes is simply hearing another person's story. This story of overcoming challenge can be the perfect gift to remind us that there is always a path out of our own suffering. It also normalizes the situation. When we hear that another person has struggles, it reminds us that we aren't failing at life. Everyone encounters adversity.

PAUSE AND FREEDOM

The pause holds power, both physically and mentally. This pause is where our freedom exists. It's what creates the space that lets us witness our experiences. Without this pause, we are simply a slave to the old mental programs that have been passed down to us through our family and culture. We are dragged down by the reptilian part of the brain, which has the single perspective of survival at the detriment of everything else.

> *"Now and then it's good to pause in our pursuit of happiness, and just be happy."*—*Guillaume Apollinaire*

But we are capable of so much more than that, as the following story illustrates. A military officer spent a significant amount of time fighting in wars overseas, and like many veterans, when he returned home he suffered from posttraumatic stress syndrome. A part of him knew that meditation and mindfulness were ways to reclaim his true self—the part of him that had been buried by the horrors of war.

After several months of a consistent meditation practice, he was in a grocery store. With only a couple of items in hand, he was about to jump into the express checkout lane when a woman holding a baby cut him off at the last second. He could feel his body gripping as the stress hormones flooded the blood stream. Thoughts began to race through his head: "How could she be so disrespectful? Just because she has a baby doesn't mean she's entitled!" To make matters worse, as the woman proceeded to unpack her grocery items, it was apparent she was over the allotted express lane amount. Being a military officer, he was used to rules. In fact, in his line of work, following rules could be a matter of life or death. As he began to count the number of items he became angrier. Every item beyond the 15 took his inner rage up another level. His heart rate sped up, his body temperature rose, his mouth dried up, and his hands became clammy.

Then something remarkable happened. His meditation practice kicked in. He noticed all these stormy biological warning signs wreaking havoc through his being. Then he paused and came back to his breath, smoothing it out. He had learned that when you shape your breath, you shape your mind. The internal storm dramatically dissipated from his body. Neurologically, he shifted from the limbic brain to the higher brain. He became free in that moment from the trauma of war and could begin to see clearly the beauty in front of him.

The customer handed the baby over to the checkout clerk, who lit up with joy. The officer thought to himself, "Why did I get so upset? I'm not even in a hurry, and even if I were, how are an extra two or three minutes going to hurt?" The happy baby was handed back to the customer, and she left the store.

All in the span of a few minutes, this officer had experienced everything from disbelief, to rage, to a moment of awakening, to empathy, and then to compassion. As his couple of items scanned through, he smiled at the check-out clerk and said, "That was one beautiful child."

The woman's eyes welled up with tears and she said, "That was my son. His father lost his life in war. Every day my mother brings my son in to see me once or twice to say hello. Since losing my husband, I've had to work two full-time jobs to pay the bills and haven't gotten to see my son much. Those moments when he comes in are the happiest of my day."

We never know what another person's story is. We never know what challenges other people are moving through. It's easy to jump to conclusions and to create stories in our head, but often this becomes a barrier to discovering the reality. Fortunately, this officer had a practice he could rely on. His ability to restore his calm saved him and the family from further suffering. Your yin yoga practice reinforces your ability to find this kind of freedom. As you can see, the benefits of yoga are bigger than becoming physically flexible.

Just the other day, I was between teaching two classes and had a tiny window of time to eat dinner. I went to a local health food store, grabbed food to go, and then sat in my car to eat. In the middle of shoveling rice, mung dhal, and steamed veggies down my throat, I saw a homeless guy lurking around my car. It was dark and he was yelling gibberish and hitting a wall. Out of nowhere, he spun around and caught me looking at him. He then jumped in front of my car, wild eyed and ragged. For a few seconds, we locked eyes.

Suddenly, he blurted out, "What time is it?!" After taking a couple of seconds to compute his question, I looked at the clock and then carefully responded, "It's 6:50." His head swung erratically to his left and then swung back to face me, and he venomously yelled, "What? What did you say?" I was somewhat scared. But my yoga practice came through. Although I experienced some fear, greater than that was a feeling of strength and courage. I began to feel a deep compassion for this human being in front of me. I couldn't help but feel the tremendous pain and suffering this soul must have endured. I felt a loving awareness flood through me like a purple dye permeating a vessel of water.

From this newfound place, I kindly reanswered his question, "It's 6:50." In a flash, all the rage in the homeless man had been erased. For a few moments we both existed together, inseparable, in a mysterious state of wonder. We were two humans, on the same plane and same level, having a weird but magical moment. A light gleamed from his eyes, and a smile manifested itself on his face. This triggered a warm smile on my face. In a voice, sweet and pure, this beautiful man said, "Oh, thank you."

After a short pause, he tenderly asked, "Hey, would you like to go to Taco Bell with me?" To say that I was caught off guard is an understatement. Nobody had ever invited me on a dinner date to Taco Bell. Once I composed myself, I said, "Thank you for the offer, but I have to go to work." We waved goodbye and as we parted ways, I couldn't help but think that this man appeared to be isolated and just needed a friend, somebody he could share a meal with at Taco Bell. The loving awareness and compassion that we gain from our yoga practice has the tremendous power to spin the micro moments of life from suffering to beauty and joy.

SEEING THE LIGHT

Take refuge within your yoga practice. Your yoga and spiritual practice provides illumination. The light of wisdom dispels the darkness of ignorance. This is illustrated in the story of a Taoist master instructing his students to do special practices at the first sign of light. The students awoke and as they were about to begin their teacher's instruction, they realized they were unsure what the first sign of light meant. They returned to their teacher and asked, "How do we know that we've seen the light? Is it when we overlook the valley and we can see the difference between an oak tree and an olive tree? Is that how we know that we've seen the light?" The master replied, "No." The students then inquired, "How about when we look out over the hills and we can see the difference between a dog and a sheep. Is that how we know that we've seen the light?" Patiently, the master answered, "No, try again." Trying to solve the puzzle, the students finally said, "I think we have it! Is it the moment when the dawn of light shoots out beyond the horizon? Is that how we know that we've seen the light?!" The master then said, "I'm sorry, no, that is not how you know you've seen the light." He continued, "You will know that you've seen the light when a stranger walks up to you and you look into their eyes and realize that the same spirit that exists inside of them is the same spirit that exists inside of you. That's how you know that you've seen the light. Until then, you are living in darkness."

On one level, we are all so different. We have different bodies, skin colors, genders, ages, nationalities, and religious beliefs, and we have all moved through different life experiences. However, on another level we are all the same. We are all one, connected through the tree of life and governed by the same laws of the Tao. The Tao says everything is born, everything lives, and everything dies. No human and no form of life escapes this.

Maybe if humanity starts looking at all the ways that we are united instead of all the ways that we are divided, a wave of transformation could take place on a colossal scale. For this deep healing to take place, the change needs to happen within our own bodies, minds, and hearts. Guess what does that? Yes, of course, your yoga practice!

As long as you live separated from the Tao, you will never be free. You will never contribute to a global awakening this is possible right now. It starts by becoming still. When you get into a yin yoga pose, that is when sensations, memories, and emotions start to surface from the depths of the connective tissue and from the depths of the heart and mind. Sometimes what comes up is fear. In fact, often when we are suffering, it's because we are trapped by fear. In some traditions, they call it the body of fear or the small self. Mythologist Joseph Campbell dedicated his life to the message of the hero's journey. The hero in every story must move through their biggest fears to become their greatest selves. As he poetically put it, "The cave that you fear to enter holds the treasure that you seek." To be all that you are capable of being, you must recognize and address your fears. This, of course, isn't easy, and that's why you have people with so much busyness in their lives. All the yang-type activity is a distraction from the reality of what people are dealing with. They would rather check out and numb out than face their own uncomfortable thoughts and situations.

LETTING GO

The Tao teaches us the courage of letting go. My meditation teacher, Jack Kornfield, says "Fear is often excitement holding its breath." At some point, you must have the courage to indulge in a full exhalation and give yourself the permission to let go. Let go of the fear, let go of the anger, and let go of the grief. Through this letting go, deep realization is possible. The following story provides an illustration of this.

A man sent a letter to the Internal Revenue Service (IRS). For those of you who live outside of the United States, the IRS is the government's tax collection agency. The following is his letter.

> Dear IRS Tax Agent,
>
> For the last several months I have not been able to sleep at night. The reason for this sudden insomnia is because I cheated on my tax report. Enclosed you will find a check for $2,000.
>
> P.S. If I still can't sleep at night I will send you a check for the rest later.

This is a funny and fascinating glimpse into the psychology of what goes on inside of people's minds: Let me let go of just enough so that I can deal with my own guilt. The question becomes why not just write a check for the entire amount, clear the slate, and fully let go? In the words of the legendary meditation teacher, Achaan Chah, "If you let go a little, you will have a little peace. If you let go a lot, you will have a lot of peace. If you let go completely, you will know complete peace and freedom" (Kornfield and Bretier 1985, 73). The time to become free is now.

You always have this choice. You are empowered to make choices today that can positively shape your destiny. Despite the challenges of the past, never underestimate the power of now. By shifting your thoughts and beliefs and then acting with clear intention, you can change your life. You can even change the world!

Feeding the Wolf

In the Native American tradition is a story about a grandfather sitting around a camp fire one evening with his two grandchildren. With the moon illuminating the sky and the wood crackling in the fire, the grandfather tells the story of two wolves fighting. It's bigger than a fight, it's an epic battle. The grandfather explains that one wolf is symbolic of the ego and represents anger, fear, guilt, resentment, jealousy, and ignorance. The other wolf is symbolic of spirit and represents love, courage, kindness, generosity, and wisdom. When the grandkids ask, "Which wolf wins the battle?" the grandfather replies, "The one that you feed the most!"

Every time you get onto your yoga mat and every time you sit on your meditation cushion, you are feeding your good wolf. The more you practice and the more you bring your practice into the world, the stronger that good wolf becomes. The things you feed become stronger and the things you starve become weaker. So, which wolf have you been feeding? Be honest with yourself: Which wolf have you been feeding? If you haven't been feeding your good wolf, then make the decision, from the depth of your being, to make the switch now. You got this and I believe in you.

Once your good wolf becomes strong, take it a step further and start feeding the good wolf within all the people you know. Feed the good wolf within your kids, family, coworkers, community members, strangers, and especially your enemies. This is how it works. When you transform your internal environment, you will transform your external environment.

It won't always be easy and that's OK. Sometimes you will be successful and other times you will fail. There is no need to worry about being perfect. Imperfections are woven into the fabric of our humanity. If you want to perfect something, work at perfecting your compassion, work at perfecting your love.

GIFT OF SPACE

Anytime you feel consumed by negativity it's because you have lost space. You have become entangled within the twists and turns of life. This is why your yoga practice is so important. It will provide the gift of space within your body, mind, and heart. Isn't this why we feel so good after yoga practice? The Buddha used the metaphor of salt and water. Imagine that you have a tablespoon of salt, and the salt represents negativity; if you pour that tablespoon of salt into a cup of water, then the cup of water becomes polluted with negativity. However, if you take that same tablespoon of salt and you pour it into a big, spacious lake, the vastness of the lake easily diffuses the salt, and the lake remains pure.

Your yin yoga practice brings that spacious quality into your entire being. You will rarely sweat the small stuff. You will snap at your kids and spouse less often. This spaciousness will create an opening for the Tao to flow.

How many amazing gifts are you missing out on because you are too busy trying to get somewhere?

The Tao is all around you. Even in the darkest of hours, the Tao is there to be unearthed. The Tao and nature and science are all one and the same. As the nature of the Tao flows, your joy and happiness grow. Joanna Macy, famed environmentalist and ecologist says, "To be alive in this beautiful, self-organizing universe—to participate in the dance of life with senses to perceive it, lungs that breathe it, organs that draw nourishment from it – is a wonder beyond words" (2003, 75).

Recently, one morning, I went to the beach with my two kids. My daughter was farther out in the ocean, body surfing. My little dude and I were playing around on the beach, half in sand, half in the water. Next to us I noticed a family that had just put their belongings down. The family consisted of an elderly couple in their late 80s or perhaps even early 90s being supported by a couple in their 50s or 60s. They didn't bring any of the typical things you see people with at the beach: no chairs, umbrellas, blankets, or even a single towel. The older couple hobbled near us in the water, still wearing their pants and undershirts. It was obvious they had very little money.

By this point, the family was becoming the object of attention to everyone on the beach that warm, sunny July day. The old man was permanently bent over and his knees were locked up. I doubt he had ever done a second of yoga in his life. Because he was frail and elderly, a part of me was concerned for his safety as the younger man supported him and they walked into the water. Sure enough, a wave came in and knocked the old man down. I held my breath in fear, watching the old man's expression after the fall. Expecting him to demand to be dragged to safety, I was surprised when the old man let out a roar of laughter that spread across the beach. Not only was he lacking typical beach paraphernalia, but he also didn't have any teeth.

This process of getting up, getting knocked down by a wave, and then laughing hysterically happened too many times to count. This beautiful old man and his family gave us all a huge gift. He taught us that when life knocks you down, you laugh and get back up. He taught us that real happiness doesn't come from owning things (not even your teeth!), it comes from your relationships. He had his wife and kids, and that meant the world to him. He taught us that no matter how close to death you are, joy exists in the present moment.

This family's joy was contagious and their light spread to all of us. My son and I played more, fell down more, and laughed more. My daughter caught a great wave. Even the dolphins came swimming by next to that Santa Monica beach. In that moment, we were all swimming in the Tao!

"Fishes are born in water. Man is born in the Tao."
—Chuang Tzu

A FINAL MESSAGE

As we wrap things up, I want to thank you for joining me on this journey of yin yoga. Take what works and leave behind what doesn't. Although I've been around the yoga block a few times, my perspective is incredibly limited. I'm sure there are many experts out there with more knowledge on the topics that we covered. I'm just sharing from my experience. But that experience is limited, and I know that. My hope is that going through this experience together—the history, knowledge, science, conversations, practices, stories, and quotes—has become more than just a book. This is why I asked my editor to call it *A JOURNEY Into Yin Yoga*. My intention is to create an environment for your personal wisdom to emerge. May your yin yoga practice always be there to guide you down your path of awakening.

If you don't mind, I would like to leave you with one last story before we officially part ways. After several years of study, a student was sent out into the forest alone by his teacher. The teacher instructed the student to report how his yoga practices were coming along. The plan was to send a progress note every several months via carrier pigeon. (This was way before text messages, emails, and tweets.) So, the student found a suitable hut and spent most hours of the day doing his spiritual practices. After several months had passed, as the teacher had requested, the student sent out the first letter. The teacher eagerly opened it and it read, "Dear teacher, today as I was meditating, my body dissolved into nothingness. I became pure white light. With my eyes closed and with my eyes open I see nothing but this light. I am happy to report I am now enlightened!" The teacher frowned, crumpled up the note, and threw it into the trash. The student thought it was strange that he never heard from his teacher, but he continued to be diligent in his practice. After several more months had passed, he sent his second note. Upon its arrival,

Bryan Kest

Bryan Kest started practicing yoga when he was 15 years old and has been practicing ever since. A yoga teacher for more than three decades, he is the creator of power yoga, a unique workout for the body, mind, and spirit. He is owner of the world-famous Santa Monica Power Yoga.

T.E. First of all, I wanted to say that one of my first yin yoga experiences was taking your world-famous LSD class. For people who are unfamiliar, what does LSD stand for?

B.K. Long, slow, and deep. That's where we got the name; it was just a description of the class. It's long. It's slow. And it's insanely deep. This class will get you more "stoned" than any other class you could possibly do. It is the ultimate drug. You leave LSD flying! Like it's not safe to drive after that class; it's not even good to talk. [laughter]

T.E. How did LSD come to be?

B.K. I had broken my shoulder mountain biking, and I still wanted to do yoga. So, I laid on the floor, I spread my legs open, and I fell forward. I just stayed in the poses, and that's where it came from. I stayed down there in that practice for, I don't know, two or three hours. When I was done, I honestly never felt more stoned in my entire life than after that practice. I knew I was onto something that was really cool. This predated yin yoga. Whoever created yin yoga hadn't released it out into the world yet. No one had ever heard of yin yoga at that time. Now, it's really, really popular for a lot of good reasons.

T.E. Being one of the most traveled teachers on the planet, are you seeing a greater demand for yin yoga?

B.K. Yeah. Yin yoga is becoming as equally popular as the most popular yoga out there now. When you talk to the studio owners, they're telling you their yin classes are packed. There is no doubt yin yoga has swept over the yoga world and it's here to stay and it's beneficial and people love it. You can easily make an argument that says, "What we all really need to do is slow down." "Oh, no! I don't want to [expletive deleted] slow down because if I slow down, then I have to feel how busy I am, and that's going to be uncomfortable. I'm going to feel my anxiety, and my nervous energy, and my antsiness. I don't want to feel that, so I'm just going to do busy yoga, right?" So, the argument is that busy people need to do slow yoga to balance out their busyness. Yin yoga is more aligned with accomplishing wellness rather than accomplishing vanity. That's important, too, because that vanity is dominated by fear. Any action that's coming from fear, you're not going to have good results.

T.E. What's your favorite yin yoga pose?

B.K. Two of them just popped into my head. One is a 10-minute forward bend (caterpillar), not that you'll see me there a lot. [laughter] The other one is a simple double pigeon (fire log).

T.E. Do you have a least favorite yin yoga pose?

B.K. Yes and no. The truth is no, because you can always tone any pose down to fit you. But that frog pose is pretty brutal! [laughter]

T.E. I know you are a fellow fan of Bruce Lee, who was inspired by the Tao. Do you have a favorite Bruce Lee quote?

B.K. "Become like water my friend," was one of his quotes, be able to move with things instead of standing in their way. If you're stuck on one way, then you might not be open to all these possibilities that are opening all around you. I heard that he brought modern boxing techniques into kung fu. Of course, all the gurus criticized him because he was perverting it. Now, he's worshiped as an innovator. And yoga has evolved over 4,000 or 5,000 or 6,000 years. It's not supposed to stop evolving. And we, you, me, anybody reading your book, they're part of that evolution. So, we have to encourage people to be creative and to trust their uniqueness and allow this to keep growing and expanding!

the teacher opened it to read, "Dear teacher, I no longer need to eat food or even drink water. [Never advised by the way!] I now live off of nothing but sunlight and the moisture in the air. On top of this great achievement, when I meditate I can astral travel through all my past lives at will!" The teacher wasn't having any of this and once again crumpled up the note and threw it into the trash.

Although the student still hadn't heard from his teacher in well over a year, he had made a pledge and continued to remain disciplined. He carried on with his practices and, as promised, sent a third note to the teacher. It read, "Dear teacher, just this morning I was chanting the sacred sound when I felt a rumbling sensation in my pelvic area. The rumbling became so strong that my body began to shake violently like an earthquake. Before I knew it, a lightning bolt of kundalini shot up my spine, lifting me off the ground so fast and so furiously that my head busted through the roof of my hut. As I levitated in midair for what must've been days, the secrets of the universe were revealed to me. I am happy to report I am now immortal!" The teacher in a state of disgust tore up the letter and stormed off absolutely furious. After the third note, almost a year passed and the teacher hadn't heard from the student. The teacher sent a letter to the student reminding him of his promise and obligation to keep sending progress reports. After a couple of weeks another letter from the student had arrived. This time it read, "Forget you. You are not my teacher and I don't need you anymore!" A huge smile spread across the teacher's face. This time he saved the note, put a beautiful frame around it, and hung it on the wall. The teacher had done his job. The student was no longer dependent; he was empowered!

Many blessings,

Travis Eliot

GLOSSARY

ahimsa—Nonviolence.

aparigraha—Nongrasping.

asana—A physical posture.

asteya—Nonstealing.

autonomic nervous system (ANS)—The system that automatically controls heart activity, blood pressure, breathing, intestinal activity, temperature regulation, and multiple other functions. Sometimes called the subconscious nervous system.

bandhas—Locks, or energy seals, that help control, contain, and harness prana and that boost the potency of yoga techniques. They are often used in yoga postures and pranayama.

bhakti yoga—The path of love and devotion.

bone—A dense type of connective tissue that protects organs, produces red and white blood cells, stores minerals, and provides support and structure for the body.

brahmacharya—Celibacy.

cartilage—A firm but flexible tissue made predominantly of protein fibers that protects the ends of long bones at the joints.

cell—The building block of life.

cell membrane—The sheath that surrounds the cell and contains the cytoplasm; defined in new biology as the brain of the cell.

chakras—The seven wheels or vortexes of energy that run through the central channel of the spine.

chi—The Taoist word for source energy or life force.

collagen—The main component of fascia. Incredibly strong, it strengthens blood vessels, keeps the skin strong, and helps build tissue by facilitating the role of fibroblasts.

connective tissues—The tissues connecting, supporting, and binding the body structures together. These include tendons, ligaments, bones, cartilage, joints, and fascia.

cytoplasm—The semifluid substance between the nuclear membrane and the cell membrane where the organelles (the cell's organs) are located.

cytoskeleton—A scaffolding-like structure that gives the cell its shape and structure.

dharana—The first stage of meditation; involves focus and concentration.

dhyana—Meditation, or total absorption into the object that is being focused on.

elastin—A highly elastic protein found in the connective tissue. After tissues in the body are stretched or contracted, elastin returns the tissues to their original shape.

extracellular matrix (ECM)—The connective tissue, ground substance, and interstitial space of the body.

fascia—A type of connective tissue enveloping the bones, muscles, and organs.

fibroblast—A type of cell that builds collagen; it is the most common type of cell in the connective tissue of animals. The primary function of fibroblasts is to maintain the structural integrity of connective tissues by secreting materials that create the extracellular matrix.

gunas—Subtle qualities underlying all creation.

hatha yoga—The path of using physical postures and breathing techniques as a way of balancing the solar and lunar energies.

hyaluronic acid (HA)—A type of fluid that fills the space between the fibers and cells of the bodily tissues; it is nature's moisturizer.

integral membrane proteins (IMPs)—The gates and channels embedded in the cell membrane that link the individual cell to its surroundings.

integrins—A type of IMP that links the cytoskeleton to the extracellular matrix. Facilitate important communication between the inner and outer cell.

ishvara pranidhana—Celebration of the divine.

jing—Considered in Chinese medicine to be the essence of human life.

jnana yoga—The yoga of knowledge.

joint—Where two bones join together and link the skeletal system as a whole.

kalapa—The smallest subatomic particle of physical matter.

karma yoga—The path of using thoughts, speech, and action in ways that are of service to others.

koshas—The layers or sheaths of the human being.

kundalini—The serpent-like primal energy awakened through yoga practices.

ligament—Tissue that connects bone to bone, often supporting a joint.

meditation—A heightened state of awareness that allows true nature to be experienced.

nadi—A pathway or channel that prana flows through.

neuroplasticity—The brain's ability to reorganize itself by forming new neural connections throughout life.

niyama—Codes for noble living; self-discipline and spiritual practices in relationship to ourselves.

nucleus—The part of the cell where DNA, important genetic information, is found. Conventional science holds the belief that the nucleus is the cell's brain.

parasympathetic nervous system—The part of the autonomic nervous system responsible for energy recovery, regeneration, repair, and relaxation.

Patanjali—A sage who systemized raja yoga into the eight limbs of yoga.

phase change—The point in a deep stretch, after approximately 90 seconds, at which you begin to access the deep fascia and connective tissues.

prana—The yoga word for source energy or life force.

prana vayus—The winds of vitality.

pranayama—The expansion of life force through breathing exercises.

pratyahara—The control of or withdrawal from the five senses.

raja yoga—Known as royal yoga or classical yoga; focuses on meditation and contemplation.

relaxin—A chemical produced in larger quantities during pregnancy that increases flexibility in the ligaments and can lead to overstretching.

restorative yoga—A style of yoga in which relaxed positions, supported by a variety of props, are held for long periods of time in order to switch on the parasympathetic nervous system.

samadhi—Absolute oneness.

santosha—Contentment.

satya—Truthfulness.

saucha—Purity.

svadhyaya—Self-study.

sympathetic nervous system—The part of the autonomic nervous system responsible for energy production and the body's ability to adapt to stress through fight or flight.

synovial fluid—Fluid secreted by the synovial membrane; it minimizes friction within the joint, making it easier for bones and cartilage to move past each other.

Tao—The way; a road, channel, or path.

Taoism—A philosophical path whose roots date back to around 550 BCE in China.

tapas—Purification.

tendon—A tough band of dense, white, fibrous connective tissue that joins a muscle to a bone.

tradak—The meditation practice of gazing at a candle flame.

Vedas—Sacred scriptures from India.

vipassana—A meditation technique taught by the Buddha; used to see things as they really are.

yama—Refers to ethics, integrity, and how yoga is practiced in daily living in relation to others.

yang—A Taoist concept representing light.

yin—A Taoist concept representing shade.

yin yoga—A system of passive floor poses held for long periods of time; used to maintain healthy connective tissues.

yoga—From the Sanskrit root word *yuj*, which means to yoke or to unite.

BIBLIOGRAPHY

Alter, M. 2004. *The Science of Flexibility*. Champaign, IL: Human Kinetics.

American Cancer Society. 2016. Lifetime Risk of Developing or Dying From Cancer. Accessed August 30, 2016. www.cancer.org/cancer/cancerbasics/lifetime-probability-of-developing-or-dying-from-cancer.

Avison, J.S. 2015. *Yoga Fascia Anatomy and Movement*. Edinburgh, Scotland: Handspring.

Beinfield, H., and Korngold, E. 1991. *Between Heaven and Earth*. New York, NY: Random House.

Benson, H. 2000. *The Relaxation Response*. New York, NY: Harper Collins.

Birney, B. 2016. "Joint Hypermobility Syndrome: Yoga's Enigmatic Epidemic?" Yoga International. Accessed February 20, 2018. https://yogainternational.com/article/view/joint-hypermobility-syndrome-yogas-enigmatic-epidemic.

Brook, J. 2010. *The Spinechecker's Manifesto*. Los Angeles, CA: Centaur Wisdom.

Centers for Disease Control and Prevention. 2016a. High Blood Pressure Fact Sheet. Accessed August 30, 2016. www.cdc.gov/dhdsp/data_statistics/fact_sheets/fs_bloodpressure.htm.

Centers for Disease Control and Prevention. 2016b. Women and Heart Disease Fact Sheet. Accessed August 30, 2016. www.cdc.gov/dhdsp/data_statistics/fact_sheets/fs_women_heart.htm.

Clark, B. 2012. *The Complete Guide to Yin Yoga*. Ashland, OR: White Cloud Press.

Clark, B. 2007. *Yinsights: A Journey into the Philosophy and Practice of Yin Yoga*. Createspace. www.createspace.com.

Choen, S., Janicki-Deverts, D., and Miller, G.E. 2007. "Psychological Stress and Disease." *Journal of the American Medical Association* 298 (14): 1605-1722.

Cowan, T. 2014. "What's the Real Cause of Heart Attacks?." Last modified May 20, 2014. https://articles.mercola.com/sites/articles/archive/2014/12/17/real-cause-heart-attacks.aspx.

Cruikshank, T. 2015. *Chinese Medicine and Myofascial Release Manual*. Yoga Medicine. https://yogamedicine.com.

Davidji. 2015. *destressifying*. Carlsbad, CA: Hay House.

Galitzer, M., and Trivieri, L. 2016. *A New Calm*. Columbus, OH: Gatekeeper.

Galitzer, M. and Trivieri, L. 2015. *Outstanding Health*. Los Angeles, CA: AHI.

Grilley, P. 2012. *Yin Yoga: Principles and Practice*. Ashland, OR: White Cloud Press.

Guimberteau, J., and Armstrong, C. 2015. *Architecture of Human Living Fascia*. Edinburgh, Scotland: Handspring.

Herman, J. 2013. *Taoism for Dummies*. Mississauga, ON, Canada: John Wiley and Sons.

Iyengar, B.K.S. 2005. *Light on Life*. Emmaus, PA: Rodale.

Kaminoff, L. 2007. *Yoga Anatomy*. Champaign, IL: Human Kinetics.

Kaptchuk, T. 2000. *The Web That Has No Weaver*. Chicago, IL: Contemporary.

Kharrazian, D. 2013. *Why Isn't My Brain Working?* Carlsbad, CA: Elephant Press.

Kishi, T. 2012. "Heart Failure as an Autonomic Nervous System Dysfunction," *Journal of Cardiology* (March 2012): 117-122

Kornfield, J. 2017. *No Time Like the Present*. New York, NY: Simon and Schuster.

Kornfield, Jack and Paul Bretier, comps. 1985. *A Still Forrest Pool: The Insight Meditation of Achaan Chah*. Wheaton, IL: Quest Books.

Lipton, B. 2005. *The Biology of Belief*. Carlsbad, CA: Hay House, Inc.

Macy, Joanna. 2003. *World as Lover, World As Self: Courage for Global Justice and Ecological Renewal*. Berkley, CA: Parallax Press.

Mitchell, Stephen. 2006. *Tao Te Ching*. New York, NY: Harper Collins.

Muktibodhananda, S. 1998. *Hatha Yoga Pradipika*. Bihar, India: Yoga Publications Trust.

Myers, T. 2014. *Anatomy Trains*. Edinburg, Scotland: Churchill Livingstone.

Olshansky, B. 2008. "Parasympathetic Nervous System and Heart Failure: Pathophysiology and Potential Implications for Therapy." *Circulation* 118 (August 19): 863-71.

Oschman, J.L. 2016. *Energy Medicine*. New York, NY: Elsevier.

Powers, S. 2008. *Insight Yoga*. Boulder, CO: Shambhala.

Rosen, R. 2002. *The Yoga of Breath*. Boston, MA: Shambhala Publications.

Saraswati, S.S. 1996. *Asana Pranayama Mudra Bandha*. Bihar, India: Yoga Publications Trust.

Talbott, S. 2002. *The Cortisol Connection*. Alameda, CA: Hunter House.

Williams, P.L. 1995. *Gray's Anatomy*. 38th Ed. Edinburgh, Scotland: Churchill Livingstone.

Wong, E. 2011. *Taoism: An Essential Guide*. Boston, MA: Shambhala.

Wooden, J. 2016. "The Tony Robbins Podcast – The Legendary John Wooden," interview by Tony Robbins, podcast audio, October 13, 2016. https://www.tonyrobbins.com/podcasts/legendary-john-wooden-interview-tony-robbins/.

Zukov, G. 1979. *The Dancing Wu Li Masters: An Overview of the New Physics*. New York: William Morrow and Company.

ABOUT THE AUTHOR

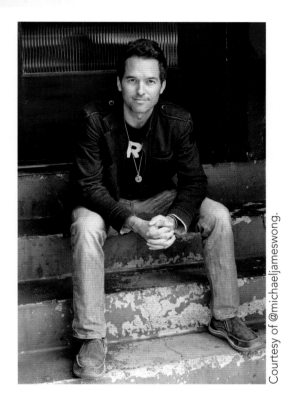

Courtesy of @michaeljameswong.

Travis Eliot is a world-renowned yoga instructor, meditation teacher, kirtan musician, and certified Ayurveda practitioner. He is the CEO of Inner Domain Media, director of Holistic Yoga Flow teacher trainings, and a member of the faculty of the prestigious Kripalu Center and the 1440 Multiversity. He teaches his signature holistic yoga flow classes in Los Angeles and in workshops and retreats around the world with an intensely dynamic style that has inspired many of today's top athletes, celebrities, and entertainers.

Eliot is the creator of the groundbreaking DVD series *The Ultimate Yogi* and the cocreator of the digital series *Yoga 30 for 30*, along with many other best-selling yoga DVDs. He is the coauthor of a comprehensive modern-day yoga book, *Holistic Yoga Flow: The Path of Practice*. His highly acclaimed chant album, *The Meaning of Soul*, debuted at number three on the iTunes world music chart. A Yoga Alliance–certified E-RYT 500 instructor, Eliot has been featured in *Yoga Journal*, *LA Yoga*, *Ayurveda and Health*, *Mantra*, *Conscious Lifestyle*, *Asana Journal*, *Self*, *Fitness Trainer*, *Access Hollywood*, and the *Huffington Post*.

Practice online with Travis at InnerDimensionMedia.com.

You read the book—now complete an exam to earn continuing education credit.

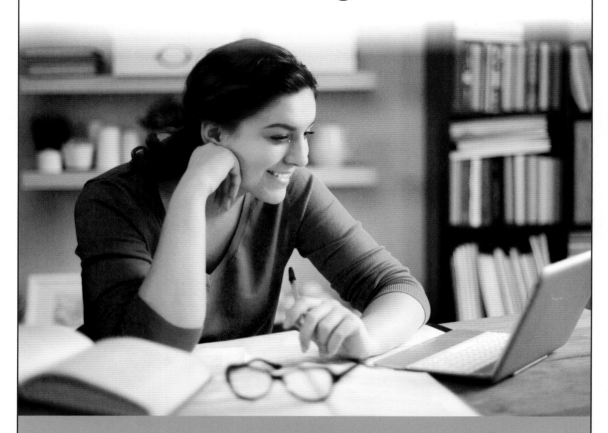

Congratulations on successfully preparing for this continuing education exam!

If you would like to earn CE credit, please visit

www.HumanKinetics.com/CE-Exam-Access

for complete instructions on how to access your exam.

Take advantage of a discounted rate by entering promo code **JYY2019** when prompted.

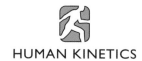